SUPER CUTE RECIPES

Glenda D. Hoppe

Copyright © 2022 by Glenda D. Hoppe

All rights reserved.

No portion of this book may be reproduced in any form without written permission from the publisher or author, except as permitted by U.S. copyright law.

Contents

1. RECIPES — 1
2. LET'S START — 5
3. Hot chocolate with cheesecake — 9
4. Breakfast smoothies with peaches and mango — 13
5. Punch for brunch — 15
6. Mimosas de pomegranate — 17
7. Bellinis apricot — 19
8. Drop doughnuts with sugar and spices — 23
9. Cinnamon buns from Grandma Billie — 29
10. Cranberry-eggnog streusel muffins — 35
11. Muffins with peanut butter and jelly — 39
12. Pumpkin bread with Nutella swirls — 43
13. Bread with apple cider — 47
14. Upside-down banana–brown butter coffee cake — 53
15. Greek scramble with cream — 57

16. Breakfast casserole made ahead of time	61
17. Sandwich with fried egg, avocado, and bacon	67
18. Breakfast pizza with sausage and scrambled eggs	71
19. Breakfast egg bake in Switzerland	75
20. Two-person o'brien egg frittata	79
21. Pancakes with pumpkin spice	85
22. Griddle cakes with bacon and corn	89
23. Crunchy cinnamon crusted french toast	95
24. Kahla–brown sugar bananas on challah french toast	99
25. Waffles with apple bacon and cider syrup	103
26. Breakfast potatoes by Susie	109
27. Almond-cranberry granola	113
28. Applesauce with maple and cinnamon	117
29. Blueberry-oatmeal breakfast bars	121
30. Beef and lentil soup in a slow cooker	127
31. Clam chowder from New England	131
32. Vegetable soup from Italy	135
33. Soup with butternut squash, pancetta, and crispy sage	139

34. Soup with roasted cherry tomatoes with macaroni and cheese — 145

35. Chilli for manly men — 149

36. Salad of grilled shrimp and vegetables with a lemon-basil dressing — 153

37. Broiled salmon with pineapple slaw — 157

Chapter One

RECIPES

BEVERAGES Pumpkin Spice Latte Recipe

Hot Chocolate with Cheesecake

Smoothies with peaches and mango for breakfast

Punch for Brunch

Mimosas with Pomegranate

Bellinis d'Apricot

PASTRIES AND BREADS

Drop Doughnuts with Sugar and Spice

Cinnamon Glazed Banana Scones

Cinnamon Rolls from Grandma Billie

Eggnog-Cranberry Muffins with Streusel

2 SUPER CUTE RECIPES

Muffins with Peanut Butter and Jelly

Bread with Nutella Swirls

Bread with Apple Cider

French Plum Coffee Cake from Grandma Amelia

Brown Butter–Banana Coffee Cake, flipped upside down

MAIN DISHES WITH EGG

Greek Creamy Scramble

Breakfast Casserole for the Next Day

Quiche with ham and Swiss cheese

Sandwich with fried egg, avocado, and bacon

Breakfast Pizza with Sausage and Scrambled Eggs

Baked Swiss Breakfast Eggs

Egg Frittata for Two by O'Brien

ADDITIONAL MAIN DISHES

Pancakes with Cinnamon Rolls

Pancakes with Pumpkin Spice

Griddle Cakes with Bacon and Corn

Pancakes that are perfect and fluffy

Crunchy Cinnamon Crust French Toast

RECIPES 3

Challah French Toast with Brown Sugar Bananas from Kahla

Waffles with Apple-Bacon and Cider Syrup

ETC. SIDES

Maple Bacon Baked in the Oven

Breakfast Potatoes Susie's

Almond-Cranberry Granola

Applesauce with Maple-Cinnamon

Blueberry Oatmeal Breakfast Bars

Chapter Two

LET'S START

WEB VEGETARIAN FAVORITE (or adaptable) GRAIN-FREE (or adaptable) NON-DAIRY (or adaptable)

latte with pumpkin spice

Approximately 1 drink Time to Prepare: 10 minutes 4 minute cook time

My husband frequently gathers a few coins and trudges down to the neighbourhood coffee shop for his fancy drink fix on fall mornings. It turns out that those dollars add up to a lot of cashola, which he uses to make his signature drink. In order to keep him at home and save money, I devised a pumpkin spice latte recipe that he adores just as much as the genuine thing.

12 gallon whole milk

1 tablespoon canned pumpkin puree, unsweetened

6   SUPER CUTE RECIPES

1 teaspoon light brown sugar, packed

1 teaspoon essence of vanilla

a quarter teaspoon of pumpkin pie spice

1 cup strong coffee, freshly made

2 tablespoons sour cream

1 teaspoon white sugar, granulated + more to taste

Optional whipped cream

Nutmeg powder

Whisk together the milk, pumpkin, brown sugar, vanilla, and spice in a glass measuring cup or microwave-safe bowl. Microwave for 1 to 2 minutes, until the milk is hot and frothy, and then remove the cup from the microwave.

Fill a tall mug or tumbler halfway with pumpkin milk. Pour in the hot coffee. Half-and-half should be added now. 1 teaspoon sugar is added. Stir, taste, and adjust the sweetness as needed.

Optional, but delicious, whipped cream and nutmeg sprinkled on top. Serve right away.

TIP Make your own pumpkin pie spice if you don't have any in your spice cabinet. Measure from there with equal parts cinnamon, ginger, allspice, and nutmeg.

Use nonfat milk and fat-free half-and-half to lighten up this dish. The drink won't be quite as rich, but the delightful pumpkin spice latte flavour will remain.

Chapter Three

Hot chocolate with cheesecake

Serves 4 people Time to Prepare: 25 minutes 5 minutes to prepare

Consider a cold, windy day with snow falling, a fire in the fireplace, and a good book and a warm beverage on the couch. Imagine that warm beverage as a rich and delicious mug of chocolate, one that will no doubt satisfy that chocolate yearning you've been feeling, and then add the whipped cream on top. This whipped cream, however, is sweetened cream cheese whipped cream, similar to that found in a cheesecake. Don't you think this Cheesecake Hot Chocolate makes a lovely picture?

CREAM WHIPPED

34 cup heavy whipping cream, chilled

3 tablespoons white granulated sugar

10 SUPER CUTE RECIPES

3 tablespoons cream cheese whipped

CHOCOLATE HEAT

4 cups low-fat milk (2% fat) (see Tips)

8 oz. chopped milk chocolate (or milk chocolate chips)

To make the whipped cream, whisk together the cream, sugar, and cream cheese in a medium mixing basin with an electric mixer. 2 to 3 minutes after lifting the beaters from the liquid, the cream should have virtually stiffened into stiff peaks. Place aside.

To make the hot chocolate, heat the milk in a medium saucepan over medium heat until it is hot to the touch, about 3 to 5 minutes. Stir in the chocolate until it melts and is fully mixed into the milk. Remove the hot chocolate from the heat and divide it among four mugs. Add a good tablespoon of whipped cream to each mug.

ADAPTABLE WITHOUT GLUTEN Use a chocolate brand that is known to be gluten-free.

TIP This recipe can be made with any type of milk; whole milk makes it richer, while skim milk makes it lighter. I utilise 2% to make anything in the centre of all of that.

Make a white hot chocolate by replacing the milk chocolate with white chocolate, and then turn it into a festive drink by adding a few drops of red, green, or pink food colouring to the hot chocolate for Christmas, Valentine's Day, or St. Patrick's Day.

Chapter Four

Breakfast smoothies with peaches and mango

Approximately 2 servings Time to Prepare: 10 minutes

On weekday mornings, getting everyone fed and out the door in a timely manner may be a little chaotic. These smoothies are loaded with fruit and yoghurt and are easy to transport. When there's a smoothie inside, tummies won't be growling for at least a couple of hours.

1 cup sliced frozen peaches

1 cup frozen mango slices

1 container vanilla yoghurt, 6 oz

a third of a cup of orange or tangerine juice + more as needed

1 teaspoon of honey

In a blender, combine all of the ingredients and blend until smooth. Simply add a bit extra juice if the smoothie appears to be too thick to combine. Serve the mixture in two glasses.

TIP Fresh peaches and mangoes can be used, but you'll need to add about 12 cup of ice cubes to get a frozen consistency.

For the peaches and mangoes, use 1 cup frozen strawberries or blueberries and 1 banana.

Chapter Five

Punch for brunch

Approximately 20 servings 15-minute prep time

This fruit juice–based punch is the one to make when you have a large group of guests over for a brunch. Your visitors can help themselves to the soup, which is served in a large bowl with a ladle. This gives you more time to prepare the rest of the meal and relieves you of the stress of having to acquire drinks for everyone. This meal is suitable for a large gathering and is suitable for children.

64 ounces pineapple juice, cold

2 cups orange juice, cold

2 cups cranberry juice, cold

1 frozen limeade concentrate 12-ounce can

1 chilled 2-liter bottle of club soda

Slices of lime and orange for garnish

Ice

Combine the liquids and limeade in a large punch bowl. Add the lime and orange slices just before serving, along with the club soda. Place the ice in a bucket and give each visitor a cup of ice and a ladleful of punch to serve themselves.

TIP Consider constructing an ice-ring for the punch bowl instead of serving ice with this punch. Combine equal parts pineapple juice, orange juice, and cranberry juice in a tiny Jello ring mould. Freeze until completely solid. To get the ring out of the pan, turn it upside down and run it under warm water until it comes loose. Float the ring in the punch bowl to keep the punch icy without watering it down like a typical ice ring.

Experiment with different juice combinations in the punch. Instead of cranberry juice, use black cherry or pomegranate juice. Use tangerine juice instead of orange juice.

Chapter Six

Mimosas de pomegranate

Approximately 6 servings 15-minute prep time

We use breakfast as an excuse to take a break from receiving gifts under the tree on Christmas morning. We have a family custom of sharing what each of us has done for charities over the past year during brunch. It's a heartwarming custom that reminds us to think about people who are less fortunate. Another custom is mimosas. They're festive, go well with brunch, and transition well into "Part Two" of the gift-giving ritual.

3 cups ice

pomegranate juice, 2 cups

2 orange juice cups

1 bottle of Champagne (750 mL)

Seeds of pomegranate

12 cup ice in each of six 12-ounce glasses Fill each glass with 13 cup pomegranate juice, 13 cup orange juice, and 12 cup Champagne. Add a few pomegranate seeds to each glass as a garnish. Serve right away.

TIPS For this recipe, use fresh orange juice.

It's simple to leave out the alcohol in this recipe if you don't want to. Simply replace the champagne with club soda.

Instead of pomegranate juice, use cranberry juice to make cranberry mimosas.

Instead of pomegranate seeds, garnish the glasses with orange wedges.

Chapter Seven

Bellinis apricot

Approximately 8 servings 15 minute prep time plus chill time 2 minute cook time

Apricots conjure up images of bright, sunny days. I like to serve this delicious apricot effervescent cocktail at a spring or summer breakfast since their obvious golden colour is sure to cheer up even the most pessimistic of individuals. The added plus is that telling your guests you're serving up fancy-schmancy "bellinis" will amaze them without requiring much effort on your part.

AN EASY SYRUP

1 cup of water

sugar (13 cup)

THE FINAL INGREDIENTS

34 cup drained canned apricot halves in syrup

1 chilled 750ml bottle of Prosecco or Champagne

Grand Marnier, 4 tablespoons (or other orange-flavored liqueur)

8 raspberries (fresh)

To make the simple syrup, put the water and sugar in a small saucepan. Bring to a boil and cook for 2 minutes, or until the sugar has dissolved. Remove the syrup from the heat, strain it into a small basin, and chill it thoroughly (about 2 hours).

In a blender, combine the simple syrup and apricots to make the apricot puree. Blend until completely smooth.

Pour 2 tablespoons of apricot puree into each of the 8 champagne glasses to make the bellinis. 13 cup Prosecco and 12 tablespoon Grand Marnier on top of each. Stir the contents of each glass gently. Serve with a raspberry on top of each drink.

ADAPTABLE WITHOUT GLUTEN Choose a gluten-free brand of apricots.

A FAST AND EASY TIP Instead of creating your own apricot puree, buy apricot nectar and use 2 tablespoons per drink.

Make your bellini taste different! Use the same recipes but substitute peaches or mangoes for the apricots, or buy canned peach or mango nectar instead.

Chapter Eight

Drop doughnuts with sugar and spices

This recipe makes 24 drop doughnuts. 30 minute prep time 12 minutes to prepare

My doughnut pan is one of those pans that collects crumbs in the back of my kitchen cupboard and wishes it had a more active existence. No special pan is required for this Portuguese-style doughnut recipe. Simply drop the batter into the hot oil, and the doughnuts rise up like magic. They're gone in a matter of seconds after a short roll in seasoned sugar. Anyone interested in a doughnut pan?

DOUGHNUTS

4 to 5 cups vegetable or canola oil

1 cup of liquid

4 tablespoons salted butter (12 stick)

SUPER CUTE RECIPES

1 tablespoon white granulated sugar

1 teaspoon of salt

1 cup flour (all-purpose)

a dozen big eggs

1 teaspoon essence of vanilla

SUGAR WITH SPICES

12 cup white granulated sugar

1 teaspoon cinnamon powder

12 teaspoon nutmeg powder

12 teaspoon clove powder

In a medium saucepan, pour the oil. 2 to 3 inches of oil is required. Heat the oil until it reaches 360°F over medium-high heat (see Tips).

Over medium-high heat, combine the water, butter, sugar, and salt in a medium saucepan. Bring to a boil while constantly whisking. Remove the pan from the heat when the mixture reaches a boil and stir in the flour until the dough comes together. Allow the dough to cool for 5 minutes in a large mixing bowl.

One at a time, beat the eggs into the dough with an electric mixer. Continue beating for 3 to 4 minutes, or until the eggs are fully mixed into the dough and the batter is thick. Blend in the vanilla extract.

Combine the spiced sugar ingredients in a low-rimmed, wide bowl.

Drop heaping tablespoons of dough into the hot oil at a time, roughly 6 at a time. As the dough balls cook, they will puff out into rounds and roll around in the oil. With a slotted metal spoon, help them along by turning them over occasionally until golden brown on all sides, about 3 to 4 minutes. Scoop the doughnuts out of the oil and place them on a paper towel–lined dish to drain for a few minutes before transferring them to the spiced sugar bowl. Sprinkle the sugar all over the doughnuts until they are completely covered. Serve right now, or keep them warm on a dish until ready to serve. Using the leftover batter and sugar, repeat the process.

TIPS You'll need a thermometer to measure the temperature of the oil in this recipe. I prefer to use a candy thermometer that can be clipped to the pan's side.

These doughnuts are best served the same day they're cooked, but they can be stored in an airtight container for up to two days.

Instead, dust the doughnuts with powdered sugar.

cinnamon-glazed banana scones

SUPER CUTE RECIPES

Approximately 6 scones 20-minute prep time 15 minutes to prepare

You either love scones or you don't, in my opinion. Scones that are dry and cardboard-like are pretty regular fare in coffee shops. When you add frosting, they become more manageable, but never totally satisfactory. These scones I have for you will turn you become a scones connoisseur. They're as soft as they come, with a light cinnamon glaze on top, and they don't taste like cardboard.

SCONES

2 cups flour (all-purpose)

12 cup white granulated sugar

1 tablespoon powdered sugar

12 teaspoon sodium chloride

12 teaspoon cinnamon powder

6 tablespoons cold salted butter, cut into cubes

12 cup ripe banana, mashed

1 egg, big

3 tablespoons heavy cream

Dusting with more flour

ICING

DROP DOUGHNUTS WITH SUGAR AND SPICES

1 cup sifted powdered sugar

2–3 teaspoons of milk

14 teaspoon cinnamon powder

Preheat the oven to 425 degrees Fahrenheit. Using nonstick spray, coat a baking sheet.

To make the scones, whisk together the flour, sugar, baking powder, salt, and cinnamon in a medium mixing bowl. Using a pastry cutter or two knives, cut in the butter until the mixture resembles fine crumbs (alternatively, this step can be done easily by pulsing the dry ingredients and butter in the food processor).

Whisk together the banana, egg, and cream in a separate medium bowl. Using a rubber spatula, carefully incorporate the dry ingredients into the wet components. Scoop the mixture onto a floured board and lightly dust with flour. Because the dough will be slightly damp, move it around on the floured surface until it is lightly covered. Make a spherical mound out of the dough (adding more flour, as needed, to keep it from sticking to the surface).

Pat the scone dough into a 9-inch round on the prepared baking sheet, about 112 inches thick. Cut the round in half using a pizza cutter or a sharp knife, then cut through the middle twice more to make 6 wedges. Pull each wedge away from the centre until there is about a 14-inch gap between them.

Bake for 15 to 18 minutes, or until the top is gently browned and the centre feels firm (no squishy center). Allow the scones to cool for at least 20 minutes after removing them from the oven.

Cut through the slightly cooled, precut slices with a sharp knife and carefully pull the scones apart. Allow to cool completely on a wire rack.

To make the icing, mix together the icing ingredients in a medium bowl with 2 tablespoons milk until smooth. If the icing is still too thick, add more milk until it reaches a dripping consistency. Drizzle the icing over the scones' tops. Allow at least 15 minutes for the icing to set before serving.

TIP These are best eaten the day they're cooked, but they're also good the next day if kept in a sealed container. Wrap and freeze if desired, then defrost when you're in the mood for a scone.

Substitute unsweetened pumpkin puree for the banana and add 12 teaspoon ground nutmeg, 14 teaspoon ground cloves, and 14 teaspoon ground ginger to make pumpkin scones.

Chapter Nine

Cinnamon buns from Grandma Billie

Approximately 24 rolls 45 minute prep time plus cooling and rising times Time to prepare: 25 minutes

When my family came to visit, my Grandma Billie would prepare these cinnamon rolls, and I remember eating them on Christmas morning in particular. We'd wake up and walk into the kitchen to find the counters covered in cinnamon rolls rising. Grandma preferred to ice the rolls with a simple sweet vanilla frosting. Perfect!

DOUGH

1 gallon whole milk

12 cup vegetable shortening

1 0.25-ounce active dry yeast packet

12 cup warm water (between 105 and 110 degrees Fahrenheit)

three huge eggs

1/2 cup white granulated sugar

1 tblsp. salt

5–6 cups flour (all-purpose)

FILLING

3/4 cup salted butter (1 1/2 sticks) at room temperature

1 cup white granulated sugar

1 cup light brown sugar, packed

2 teaspoons cinnamon powder

GLAZE

1 cup sifted powdered sugar

whole milk, 1 to 2 teaspoons

1/2 teaspoon extract de vanille

To make the dough, heat the milk and shortening in a small saucepan until the shortening has melted. Remove the pan from the fire and set it aside to cool to a lukewarm temperature, about 30 minutes.

Dissolve the yeast in the warm water in a small bowl and set away until the yeast bubbles (see Tips).

1 to 2 minutes in the bowl of a stand mixer, whisk the eggs, sugar, and salt until frothy. Combine the milk and yeast mixtures. (If you don't have a stand mixer, see Tips.)

Change the mixer's beaters to a dough hook and gradually add the 5 cups flour, scraping down the sides of the bowl as needed, until the flour is well integrated. The dough should form into a ball and begin to lift from the mixing bowl's bottom. As needed, add more flour a bit at a time until the dough forms a ball and is no longer sticky. Allow the dough hook to do its work and knead for around 5 minutes.

Using nonstick spray, coat a medium bowl. Scrape the dough into the basin and turn it over, allowing the oil to coat all sides. Cover the basin with a clean dish cloth and place it in a warm location to rise for 1 to 2 hours, or until nearly doubled. Nonstick spray two 9 x 13-inch baking pans. Place aside.

Punch down the risen dough and place it on a lightly floured surface to add the filling. With the long side facing you, roll out the dough into a large rectangle, 14 to 12 inch thick (adding more flour, as needed, to prevent the dough from sticking to the surface). Spread softened butter over the dough. First, evenly sprinkle the white sugar, then evenly sprinkle the brown sugar, and then evenly sprinkle the cinnamon.

Roll the dough over the filling, starting with the long side nearest to you, until you have one giant log of rolled dough.

Remove and discard the ends. Slice 1-inch-wide cinnamon rolls using a sharp knife. Carefully transfer the cut rolls to two oiled 9 x 13-inch pans. In each pan, place 12 rolls.

Here are the baking instructions: Cover the pans loosely with clean dish cloths and set them aside to rise for 1 to 2 hours, or until they've nearly doubled in size.

Baking instructions to follow later: Refrigerate the pans for up to 1 day after covering them with plastic wrap. Remove them from the fridge, remove the plastic wrap, and cover them loosely with clean dish cloths before baking. Place the pans in a warm location to rise until they've about doubled in size. Place them in a cold oven overnight (put on the light but not the heat) if you want to eat them first thing in the morning. In the morning, they should have risen and be ready to bake. Then follow the baking directions listed below.

Preheat the oven to 350°F for baking. Remove the dish cloths from the cinnamon rolls and bake for 15 to 20 minutes, or until golden brown. Remove the rolls from the oven and cool for a few minutes.

Whisk together the glaze ingredients in a medium bowl, adding just enough milk to achieve a drizzling consistency. Serve immediately with the glaze drizzled over the warm rolls.

TIPS When mixing yeast with water, the temperature of the water is critical. It's possible that too much heat will destroy the yeast. If the yeast does not bubble, your yeast is most likely no longer active, and you should try again with a new packet.

If you don't have a stand mixer, beat the eggs, sugar, and salt with a standard hand mixer. Combine the milk and yeast mixtures in a mixing bowl. Then, one cup at a time (5 cups total), whisk in the flour until completely combined. Transfer the dough to a floured surface and knead it for 5 to 8 minutes, until it comes together to form a ball and is no longer sticky, adding flour as needed. Continue with the rising instructions.

If desired, add raisins or nuts to your cinnamon rolls. Because we're not a raisin or nut family, I usually leave those out.

Chapter Ten

Cranberry-eggnog streusel muffins

Approximately 14 to 16 muffins 15-minute prep time Time to prepare: 20 minutes

When the holidays arrive in the fall, I am absolutely fascinated of all things eggnog. I prefer to appreciate the flavour of eggnog by baking with it rather than drinking it straight from the carton, which regrettably goes straight to my hips. These eggnog-flavored muffins are topped with a simple sugar-and-nut streusel, and they're sure to please eggnog fans.

BATTER MUFFIN

214 cup flour (all-purpose)

1 tablespoon powdered sugar

1 cup granulated white sugar + 2 teaspoons granulated white sugar, divided

¾ cup low-fat or standard eggnog

⅓ cup melted salted butter

2 eggs, big

1 teaspoon extract (almond, vanilla, or eggnog)

1 cup roughly chopped frozen cranberries (see Tips)

TOPPING STREUSEL

½ cup white granulated sugar

½ cup flour (all-purpose)

4 tablespoons salted butter, slightly softened (½ stick)

½ cup chopped pecans, if desired

Preheat the oven to 400 degrees Fahrenheit. Using nonstick spray, coat 16 muffin cups.

To make the muffin batter, whisk together the flour and baking powder in a medium mixing dish. Place aside.

Whisk together 1 cup sugar, eggnog, butter, eggs, and extract in a large mixing basin. Stir in the dry ingredients until barely mixed. Toss the cranberries with the remaining 2 tablespoons sugar in a separate bowl. Incorporate the mixture into the muffin batter.

To make the streusel topping, combine the streusel ingredients in a medium bowl using a pastry cutter or a fork until crumbly.

Fill the muffin cups two-thirds full with batter. 1 tablespoon of the streusel topping should be placed in each muffin cup. Bake for 18–22 minutes, or until a toothpick inserted in the centre comes out clean. Allow 10 minutes for the muffins to cool on a wire rack before removing them from the pan.

TIP Have you only got fresh cranberries? Place them on a rimmed baking sheet and place them in the freezer until solid. Chopping frozen cranberries is much easier.

Instead of a streusel topping, drizzle these muffins with an eggnog glaze! 14 cup powdered sugar, 1 tablespoon eggnog, and a pinch of nutmeg, sprinkled Drizzle the glaze over the muffins' tops.

Chapter Eleven

Muffins with peanut butter and jelly

Approximately 12 muffins 20-minute prep time Time to prepare: 20 minutes

The best part about having a child in the house is that peanut butter and jelly are constantly on hand. Okay, fine... Maybe it's not the "greatest" thing, but it's certainly a benefit of having children. I've turned everyone's favourite breakfast sandwich into muffins. In the middle of the peanut buttery cake, a large dollop of your favourite jam is dumped.

123 cup flour (all-purpose)

12 cup light brown sugar, packed

1 tablespoon powdered sugar

1 tablespoon salt

¾ cup milk

SUPER CUTE RECIPES

12 cup peanut butter (creamy) (see Tips)

13 cup vegetable or canola oil

1 egg, big

12 tsp vanilla extract

12 cup strawberry jam (see Variations!)

Preheat the oven to 350 degrees Fahrenheit. Using nonstick spray, coat 12 muffin cups.

Whisk together the flour, sugar, baking powder, and salt in a medium mixing basin. Place aside.

Whisk together the milk, peanut butter, oil, egg, and vanilla in a separate medium bowl. Combine the wet and dry ingredients in a mixing bowl and stir just until mixed.

Fill each muffin cup with roughly 2 teaspoons of batter. Top each cup of batter with a heaping tablespoon of jam. Then, on top of the jam, pour around 2 teaspoons of batter. Any leftover batter should be divided evenly among the muffin cups.

Bake for 20 to 25 minutes, or until the muffins are firm to the touch and have risen in the centre.

TIP If you choose a natural-style peanut butter for this recipe, make sure it's a creamy, no-stir variety. To make lovely, moist, and soft muffins, you'll need the oils found in peanut butter.

MUFFINS WITH PEANUT BUTTER AND JELLY

For this recipe, use your favourite jam variety. The blackberry is a particularly good strawberry alternative.

Make almond butter muffins by replacing the peanut butter with a creamy, nonstir kind of almond butter.

Chapter Twelve

Pumpkin bread with Nutella swirls

1 loaf of bread 20-minute prep time 1 hour and 15 minutes to prepare

I've been making a basic pumpkin bread recipe for years, and during the holidays, I give away dozens of loaves to family and friends. It's far from ordinary. It's juicy, spicy, hearty, and just right. When you swirl Nutella into this bread, though, it becomes even more delicious. It's the hip and cool version of my original pumpkin bread, in my opinion.

12 cup flour (all-purpose)

1 teaspoon bicarbonate of soda

a quarter teaspoon of baking powder

1 teaspoon cinnamon powder

12 teaspoon nutmeg powder

12 teaspoon clove powder

12 teaspoon allspice powder

12 teaspoon sodium chloride

12 cup white granulated sugar

12 cup vegetable or canola oil

2 eggs, big

1 cup pumpkin puree, unsweetened

1 cup of water

Nutella (14 cup) (or another chocolate hazelnut spread)

Preheat the oven to 350 degrees Fahrenheit. Using nonstick spray, coat a 9-inch loaf pan (see Tips).

Whisk together the flour, baking soda, baking powder, spices, and salt in a medium mixing basin. Place aside.

Combine the sugar, oil, and eggs in a large mixing bowl with an electric mixer. Mix in the dry ingredients until they are completely combined. Mix in the pumpkin puree and water until all of the ingredients are thoroughly blended.

Place the Nutella in a medium dish and microwave for about 20 seconds to soften it. Stir in 13 cup of the pumpkin batter with the Nutella until well combined.

Half of the pumpkin batter should be poured into the prepared pan. Half of the Nutella batter should be poured over the pumpkin batter (little spoonfuls about 1 inch apart). Pour the remaining pumpkin batter on top of the Nutella, then top with the remaining Nutella batter. Gently swirl the batters together with a knife a few times.

1 hour and 15 minutes in the oven, or until a toothpick inserted in the centre comes out clean. Cool for at least 15 minutes in the pan before turning out onto a wire rack to finish cooling.

TIPS This recipe yields a substantial loaf of bread. If you use a loaf pan that is smaller than 9 5 inches, you'll want to bake a few muffins with the leftover batter.

This bread can be frozen. Cover with plastic wrap and then foil once it has cooled. Keep frozen until ready to consume. It keeps for several weeks in the freezer.

To prepare the classic version of my pumpkin bread, leave off the Nutella entirely.

By omitting the Nutella and replacing it with 1 cup small chocolate chips, this recipe becomes Chocolate Chip Pumpkin Bread.

Chapter Thirteen

Bread with apple cider

1 loaf of bread (12 servings) 15-minute prep time Time to prepare: 50 minutes

I hope you're fortunate enough to reside in an area with apple trees. Autumn apple harvesting is one of the nicest family activities available. Apples are plucked from trees and lovingly placed in collection bags by the children. It's a great time for everyone involved. Coming home with an abundance of apples and deciding what to do with them is the best part. The obvious answer is applesauce, but apple cider bread should be a close second.

2 cups flour (all-purpose)

1 teaspoon powdered baking soda

1 teaspoon bicarbonate of soda

1 tblsp. salt

SUPER CUTE RECIPES

1 teaspoon cinnamon powder

12 teaspoon clove powder

⅔ cup granulated white sugar

⅓ cup packed light brown sugar

4 tablespoons unsalted butter (12 stick) at room temperature

2 eggs, big

½ cup apple cider (or apple juice) (or apple juice)

2¼ cups peeled and cored chopped apples (approximately 3 large) (about 3 large)

1 tablespoon lemon juice, freshly squeezed

Preheat the oven to 350 degrees Fahrenheit. An 8-inch loaf pan should be greased and floured.

Sift the flour, baking powder, baking soda, salt, cinnamon, and cloves into a medium mixing basin.

1 to 2 minutes with an electric mixer, whisk the sugars and butter in a large mixing bowl until light and creamy. Incorporate the eggs until fully combined. Mix in half of the flour mixture at a time, alternating with the cider, until barely incorporated.

Toss the apples with the lemon juice in a small bowl. Add the apples to the batter and mix well.

Scoop the batter into the pan that has been prepared. Bake for 50-60 minutes, or until a toothpick inserted in the middle comes out clean. Cool for at least 20 minutes in the pan before turning out onto a wire rack to cool completely.

TIPS In this bread, I prefer to use a variety of apples. Gala, Granny Smith, Braeburn, and Jonathon types are my favourites.

This is one of those breads that tastes better the second day. It will keep for several days if stored in an airtight container or tightly wrapped.

Warm slices drizzled with hot caramel sauce can be served as a dessert.

French plum coffee cake from Grandma Amelia

Serves 18 people Time to Prepare: 25 minutes Time to prepare: 25 minutes

Every fall, my sister Susie's friend Dana (are you still with me?) brings plum coffee cake to the workplace to share. It's a recipe from her granny. I drooled as I listened to my sister describe the cake: how it looked, how it tasted, and how the entire staff at her middle school gobbled it in no time. Dana was kind enough to share the recipe with her. Dana asked Grandma, and Grandma said yes, so now we can all enjoy Grandma Amelia's French Plum Coffee Cake. It sounds sophisticated

SUPER CUTE RECIPES

with the French plums, but you can make the cake with plain plums and it will be perfect.

CAKE

1 cup white granulated sugar

8 tablespoons salted butter (1 stick) at room temperature 1 lemon zest, grated

1 big egg 1 teaspoon salt

2 cups flour (all-purpose)

2 teaspoons bicarbonate of soda

34 gallon full milk

4 tiny plums, cut in half, pit removed, and thinly sliced

STREUSEL

34 cup flour (all-purpose)

2/3 cup white granulated sugar

4 tablespoons salted butter (12 stick) melted

12 teaspoon cinnamon powder

Preheat the oven to 350 degrees Fahrenheit. Using nonstick spray, coat a 13 x 18-inch jelly-roll pan (see Tips).

To make the cake, combine the sugar, butter, and lemon zest in a large mixing bowl with an electric mixer. Combine the egg and salt in a mixing bowl.

Sift the flour and baking soda into a separate basin. A bit at a time, stir the dry ingredients into the wet components, alternating with the milk. Pour the batter into the pan that has been prepared. Arrange the plum wedges on top of the batter in rows for a beautiful effect.

To make the streusel, combine all of the streusel ingredients in a medium mixing bowl and stir until crumbly. Sprinkle the streusel topping evenly over the plums.

Bake for 25 to 35 minutes, or until a toothpick inserted in the centre comes out clean. Allow at least 20 minutes for the cake to cool before cutting and serving.

TIP A standard-size, rimmed baking sheet is a 13 x 18-inch jelly-roll pan (otherwise known as a half sheet pan). This cake will be best baked in this pan.

Make a different fruit cake with this recipe. Replace the plums with sliced nectarines or peaches.

Chapter Fourteen

Upside-down banana–brown butter coffee cake

Approximately 6 servings Time to Prepare: 25 minutes 35 minutes to prepare

I experimented with this cake recipe on a Sunday morning many moons ago. My family was looking forward to a special weekend brunch, and I was determined to cook it with brown butter… and bananas… and turn it upside down. The outcome was this dish, which was a tremendous hit with my two sons. Dare I say the three of us finished the cake in one sitting?

TOPPING

4 tablespoons salted butter (12 stick)

2 tbsp. light brown sugar, packed

2 teaspoons white granulated sugar

34 teaspoon cinnamon powder

SUPER CUTE RECIPES

1 ripe medium banana, cut (see Tips)

CAKE

4 tablespoons salted butter (12 stick) at room temperature

14 cup white granulated sugar

1 ripe banana, mashed

1 pound sour cream

1 egg, big

12 teaspoon extract de vanille

1 cup flour (all-purpose)

12 teaspoon powdered baking soda

12 teaspoon bicarbonate of soda

12 teaspoon cinnamon powder

1/8 teaspoon ginger powder

1 teaspoon of salt

Preheat the oven to 350 degrees Fahrenheit. Using cooking spray, coat an 8-inch round or square cake pan.

Melt the butter in a small saucepan over medium-low heat to make the topping. 5 to 6 minutes of stirring until the butter begins to brown. Remove the pan from the heat and pour the browned butter into it, swirling it around to coat the bottom.

UPSIDE-DOWN BANANA–BROWN BUTTER COFFEE CAKE

Combine the sugars and cinnamon in a small bowl. Over the browned butter in the skillet, sprinkle evenly. Place the banana slices on top of the sugars in an even layer.

To make the cake, cream together the butter and sugar in a medium mixing bowl with an electric mixer. Combine the banana, sour cream, egg, and vanilla in a mixing bowl.

Whisk together the flour, baking powder, baking soda, cinnamon, ginger, and salt in a separate dish. Combine the dry ingredients and stir them into the banana mixture. Pour the batter into the pan and equally distribute the bananas.

30–35 minutes in the oven, or until a toothpick inserted in the centre comes out clean. Remove the cake from the oven and loosen with a sharp knife down the pan's side. Place a serving plate on top of the pan and turn it over gently. The cake should readily release from the pan and onto the dish. If the cake needs coaxing, tap the bottom of the pan. Drizzle any leftover pan juices over the top of the cake. Serve right away.

TIP Use ripe, soft bananas with lots of brown spots, not the dead black variety.

Make an Upside-Down Brown Butter-Banana-Blueberry Coffee Cake using this cake. Instead of putting banana slices on the bottom of the pan, sprinkle blueberries on top.

Toss in some almond pieces or roasted walnuts.

Chapter Fifteen

Greek scramble with cream

Serves 4 people 20-minute prep time Time to cook: 4 to 6 minutes

This cookbook does not include omelettes, and for good reason. I simply dislike them, and I've never been particularly good at producing them. An omelette is usually all egg with very little "stuff." I start in the middle and work my way through everything excellent, but I quickly find myself with a plate full of overcooked egg scraps. What's the answer? It's a jumble. I assume that if you scramble all of that excellent omelette stuff into your eggs, you won't have any plain eggs left over.

8 eggs, big

2 teaspoons liquid

1 teaspoon lemon juice, freshly squeezed

1 tablespoon sour cream

12 cup spinach leaves, chopped

12 cup cherry tomatoes, diced

12 cup feta or goat cheese, crumbled

Optional: 1 teaspoon minced fresh chives

To taste, season with salt and freshly ground black pepper.

Whisk together the eggs, water, and lemon juice in a medium mixing basin. You want to mix the water and lemon juice into the eggs, so whisk them thoroughly. Place aside.

Spray a medium skillet with nonstick spray and heat to medium. Allow 1 minute for the cream cheese to melt in the pan, stirring it around to soften it. Give the eggs one more good stir before adding them to the hot pan. Travel them around with a rubber spatula while they cook, allowing the raw egg to move about the pan. Add the spinach, tomatoes, and cheese when the eggs are almost done, and continue to stir the eggs until the spinach has wilted and the eggs are fully cooked. Remove the pan from the heat and, if wanted, garnish with chives. Season with salt and pepper to taste right away.

TIP Try not to chop your vegetables while your eggs are cooking. This recipe is made easier by having everything chopped and ready to go ahead of time.

For a distinct flavour, mix in 12 teaspoon of freshly chopped dill with the vegetables.

GREEK SCRAMBLE WITH CREAM

Replace the feta or goat cheese with cheddar or Swiss cheese.

Add a variety of vegetables, such as softly steamed broccoli or sautéed mushrooms, zucchini, and shallots.

Chapter Sixteen

Breakfast casserole made ahead of time

Approximately 10 servings 30 minutes of prep time plus an overnight chill 1 hour and 10 minutes to prepare

For many years, my family has made various versions of this "feeds-a-large-crowd" breakfast dish. It's the ideal low-stress option for entertaining guests and family because everything is prepared the night before, and it's so good that there's rarely any leftovers. However, leftovers of this casserole are a wonderful thing.

8 cups squares of day-old French bread or focaccia (half of a 1-pound loaf)

2 teaspoons melted salted butter

8 ounces sliced kielbasa sausage, chopped into bite-size pieces

2 cups shredded sharp cheddar cheese (8 ounces)

1 cup shredded Swiss cheese, 4 oz.

8 eggs, big

12 cup low-fat milk with 2% fat

14 cup white wine, dry

2 thinly sliced entire green onions, white and light green sections

2 tablespoons Mustard dijon

cayenne pepper, 1/8 teaspoon

a quarter cup of sour cream

12 cup Parmesan cheese, freshly grated

Nonstick spray a 9 x 13-inch baking dish.

In the prepared dish, equally distribute the bread cubes and drizzle with butter. Add the meat and cheeses and mix well. Whisk together the eggs, milk, wine, green onions, mustard, and cayenne in a medium mixing basin. Cover the casserole with plastic wrap and place in the refrigerator overnight.

Refrigerate the casserole for at least 30 minutes before baking it. Preheat the oven to 350 degrees Fahrenheit.

Remove the casserole from the plastic wrap. Using nonstick spray, coat a sheet of foil and place it over the casserole, sprayed side down. 1 hour in the oven Remove the casserole from the oven, remove the foil, and top with the sour cream and Parmesan cheese. Bake for a further 10 minutes, uncovered, or until the casserole is golden brown and cooked through. Allow 15 minutes to cool before slicing and serving.

TIP I appreciate the flavour that the wine adds to the casserole, but if you don't want to use alcohol, simply add an extra 14 cup of milk.

If preferred, 8 ounces cooked and crumbled sausage can be substituted for the kielbasa.

Instead of French bread, use egg bread/challah.

In place of the cheddar-Swiss combo, a blend of Mexican shredded cheese works well in this dish.

quiche with ham and Swiss cheese

This recipe makes one 9-inch quiche. 35-minute prep time 45 minutes to prepare

I eat quiche for breakfast, lunch, and dinner, as well as late at night as leftovers. It's one of those things that always appears to me to be a wonderful supper. The best part about a quiche is that it also feels like dessert. Baked in a pie pan with a flaky crust and a creamy egg custard filling. Even though it contains broccoli, ham, and Swiss cheese, it seems like you're eating dessert. Breakfast dessert works for me.

CRUST

SUPER CUTE RECIPES

12 cup flour (all-purpose)

13 cup unsalted cold butter, cut into cubes

1/8 teaspoon nutmeg powder

1 teaspoon of salt

cayenne pepper, 1/8 teaspoon

2 tbsp ice water + additional as needed

1 teaspoon vinegar, white

FILLING

1 tablespoon extra virgin olive oil

1 cup onion, chopped (about 1 medium)

1 cup ham diced

1 teaspoon garlic, minced (1 large clove)

2 cups broccoli florets, tiny

6 eggs, big

1 cup heavy cream (whipped)

2 tablespoons brown mustard, hot

1 tablespoon salt

1/8 teaspoon white pepper, ground

6 oz. shredded Swiss cheese (112 cup)

BREAKFAST CASSEROLE MADE AHEAD OF TIME

Preheat the oven to 350°F and nonstick coat a 9-inch deep-dish pie pan.

To make the crust, pulse the flour, butter, nutmeg, salt, and cayenne together a few times in a food processor until thick crumbs form. Combine the 2 tablespoons water and the vinegar in a small bowl and slowly drip the liquid into the processor while it is running. The dough should form clumps as it rises. If required, add 12 tablespoons of icy water at a time until the dough comes together. Remove the dough from the processor and pat it into a round on a piece of plastic wrap. While you make the filling, wrap the round in plastic wrap and leave it in the refrigerated for at least 15 minutes.

To make the filling, heat the oil in a large skillet over medium heat. Cook for 3 to 4 minutes, or until the onion is softened and gently browned. Cook for another 2 minutes after adding the ham and garlic. Cook for a further 2 minutes after adding the broccoli. Turn off the heat in the pan.

Whisk together the eggs, cream, mustard, salt, and pepper in a medium mixing bowl. Place aside.

Roll out the crust between two pieces of plastic wrap into a circular about 12 inches in diameter. Remove the top layer of plastic wrap from the crust and flip it over into the prepared pie plate. Remove the last piece of plastic wrap from the crust and carefully press it into the pan, crimping the edges as desired.

Fill the crust with the cooked vegetables. On top, sprinkle the cheese. Pour over the egg custard.

Bake for 40 to 45 minutes, or until the quiche's top is golden brown and the filling has set. Allow 15 minutes to cool before slicing.

ADAPTABLE TO VEGETARIANS Leave the ham out and replace it with another cup of vegetables.

EASY AND QUICK Purchase a prepared crust and follow the recipe's instructions.

TIP Quiche keeps well in the refrigerator for 2 to 3 days. Refrigerate it after wrapping it in plastic wrap.

Cooked bacon or cooked, crumbled sausage can be substituted for the ham.

Replace the Swiss cheese with your preferred cheese or a combination of cheeses.

Quiche with sautéed mushrooms is delicious. Add them in or replace the broccoli with them.

Chapter Seventeen

Sandwich with fried egg, avocado, and bacon

Approximately 1 sandwich 15-minute prep time 10 minutes to prepare

Avocados were never on my dinner menu when I was a kid. I'm not sure if they weren't easily available in the 1970s, if they weren't fashionable, or if the ordinary housewife didn't know what to do with one. Avocados were first introduced to me in college through guacamole. Avocados are now in my grocery cart every time I go to the store, and they're not only for guacamole any longer. Avocados also go well with egg, bacon, tomato, and pepper Jack cheese in a sandwich.

2 bacon pieces

2 bread slices

1 egg, big

1 pepper Monterey Jack cheese slice

2 tomato slices

12 sliced avocado

a quarter teaspoon of lemon pepper a pinch of salt

Cook the bacon in a medium skillet over medium heat until crisp, about 6 to 8 minutes. To drain the bacon, place it on paper towels. Wipe the skillet clean.

While the egg is cooking, toast the bread in the toaster.

Spray the skillet with nonstick spray and heat to medium. Cook for 2 to 3 minutes, or until the egg white begins to turn opaque white. Flip the egg over gently with a rubber spatula. Cook the egg for a further 1 to 2 minutes, or until it is no longer raw (see Tips).

On a dish, place one slice of bread. Add the cheese on top. The fried egg should be slid onto the cheese. Combine the bacon, tomato, and avocado in a bowl. Season with salt and lemon pepper. Place the second slice of bread on top. Cut the sandwich in half with a sharp knife and serve right away.

ADAPTABLE WITHOUT GLUTEN Use a gluten-free bacon brand and gluten-free bread instead of ordinary bread.

ADAPTABLE DAIRY-FREE Remove the cheese.

ADAPTABLE TO VEGETARIANS Leave the bacon out.

SANDWICH WITH FRIED EGG, AVOCADO, AND BACON

TIP Cook the egg so that some of the yolk is still runny on the inside. When you cut it open, part of the yolk will drip into your plate, making a tasty sandwich dipping sauce!

Change up the cheese flavour or add some hot sauce to the mix.

Chapter Eighteen

Breakfast pizza with sausage and scrambled eggs

Approximately 8 slices 20-minute prep time Time to prepare: 20 minutes

Near my residence, there's a deli that specialised in pizza. The best business decision they made was to start selling breakfast pizza. It was such a tremendous hit that I decided to try to recreate it at home. This dish is quite similar to what we order from a pizza delivery service. It's a sour cream and salsa-topped sausage, egg, and cheese pizza. On lazy Sunday mornings when my guys are lying around watching football, I love to make it.

1 pound spicy pork ground sausage

6 big, lightly beaten eggs

12 teaspoon black pepper, freshly ground

Rolling out the pizza dough using all-purpose flour

pizza dough (1 pound) (see Tips)

cornmeal, 2 tablespoons

1 salsa jar (16 oz.)

2 cups shredded Mexican blend cheese (8 ounces)

Optional: 34 cup sour cream

Preheat the oven to 425 degrees Fahrenheit. Preheat the oven for 30 minutes with a pizza stone on the bottom rack. (If you don't have a pizza stone, see Tips.)

Brown the sausage in a large nonstick skillet over medium heat, tossing often, until it crumbles and is no longer pink, about 5 to 7 minutes. Place the sausage on a platter lined with paper towels. Drain and set aside. Wipe out the skillet. Whisk together the eggs and pepper in a medium mixing basin. Place aside. Roll out the dough into a 12- to 14-inch circle on a floured surface. Sprinkle cornmeal on the pizza stone and slide the dough onto it. Bake for 4 minutes, or until the crust is lightly browned and bubbling.

Cook the eggs in a lightly oiled skillet over medium heat, without stirring, until they begin to firm on the bottom, while the crust is baking. Make huge curds with a rubber spatula across the bottom of the skillet. Cook until the eggs have thickened but are still wet (do not stir constantly). Turn off the heat and set the skillet aside.

BREAKFAST PIZZA WITH SAUSAGE AND SCRAMBLED EGGS

Carefully open the oven and slide out the rack when the crust is gently browned and bubbling. Distribute the salsa equally over the half baked crust, then top with sausage, scrambled eggs, and cheese. Bake for another 8 to 12 minutes, or until the cheese has melted and the crust has turned a deep golden brown colour.

Before slicing, remove the pizza from the oven and let it cool for at least 10 minutes. If preferred, serve slices with sour cream.

TIPS Make your own pizza dough, buy prefabricated pizza dough at the store, or ask a pizza establishment to sell you a 1-pound dough ball.

Use a pizza pan or a cookie sheet instead of a pizza stone if you don't have one. Simply sprinkle the pan with cornmeal before laying the dough on it, and do not warm the pan in the oven like the stone.

Use reduced-fat sausage, egg whites, reduced-fat cheese, and low-fat sour cream to lighten up this recipe.

Make this breakfast pizza with your favourite pizza toppings! Cooked bacon, tomato, caramelised onions, various cheeses, and ham are all good options.

Chapter Nineteen

Breakfast egg bake in Switzerland

Approximately 6 servings Time to Prepare: 25 minutes 30 minutes to prepare

When the weekend arrives, my family expects something special for breakfast. I'd be delighted to create something unique for them. If we eat breakfast out, we're going to spend a lot of money and consume significantly more calories than one should consume in the morning. This baked egg casserole is one of my favourite weekend breakfasts. It's loaded with vegetables, and it provides you a lot more energy than sluggishness on a lazy weekend day.

1 tablespoon butter (salted)

1 sliced medium leek (about 34 cup)

2 cups Swiss chard, finely sliced (3 to 4 big leaves, ribs removed)

SUPER CUTE RECIPES

1 cup pear tomatoes, halved

8 eggs, big

Ricotta cheese (34 cup)

12 gallon whole milk

shredded Swiss cheese (23 cup), divided

1 tablespoon mustard (Dijon)

12 teaspoon sodium chloride

cayenne pepper (1/4 teaspoon)

Preheat the oven to 350 degrees Fahrenheit. Using nonstick spray, coat a 9-inch square pan.

Melt the butter in a medium skillet over medium heat. Cook for 2 to 3 minutes, or until the leek begins to soften. Toss in the tomatoes and Swiss chard. Cook for an additional 2 to 3 minutes, covered, until the chard has wilted. Turn off the heat and set the pan aside to cool.

Whisk together the eggs, ricotta, milk, 13 cup Swiss cheese, mustard, salt, and cayenne in a large mixing basin.

In the bottom of the prepared pan, spread the cooled vegetables. On top, pour the egg mixture.

20 minutes in the oven On top of the egg, sprinkle the remaining 13 cup Swiss cheese. Bake for another 10 minutes,

or until an inserted knife into the centre of the egg bake comes out clean.

ADAPTABLE WITHOUT GLUTEN Make sure to use a gluten-free Dijon mustard.

TIP Do all of your cutting the night before so you can make this quickly in the morning. The next day will be a breeze to prepare.

Although this egg dish is vegetarian, you can add cooked bacon, ham, or sausage to make it more interesting. You can also change up the cheese you use.

Chapter Twenty

Two-person o'brien egg frittata

Approximately 2 servings 30 minute prep time 30 minutes to prepare

After I've dropped my son off at school, I like to make a small breakfast for my husband and me every now and again. This one can even be served for lunch or dinner on occasion. There's lots of cheddar, onions, bell peppers, and bacon in this egg and potato meal. The best part is that it only serves two people, so if there are only two of you, you won't be able to overeat!

2 halved medium red potatoes

4 big, lightly beaten eggs

split 34 cup shredded cheddar cheese

1 tablespoon butter, unsalted

SUPER CUTE RECIPES

1⁄2 cup red bell pepper, diced

1⁄2 cup prosciutto or diced Canadian bacon

1⁄3 cup green onion, white and green sections finely sliced

2 minced garlic cloves

a quarter cup of sour cream

Preheat the oven to 450 degrees Fahrenheit.

Fill a small saucepan halfway with water and add the potatoes. Heat the water to a rolling boil. Cook for 10 to 15 minutes, or until the potatoes are just soft. Drain, then chop with the peel still attached.

In a mixing dish, whisk together the eggs and 1⁄4 cup of the cheese. Place aside.

Melt the butter in a 10-inch oven-safe skillet over medium heat. Cook, stirring occasionally, until the bell pepper, bacon, onion, and garlic are softened, about 5 minutes. Pour the egg mixture over and around the potatoes in the skillet, making sure they are equally distributed. Cook for 5 minutes over medium-low heat, or until almost set. 1⁄2 cup cheese remains to be sprinkled on top.

Bake for 5 minutes, or until the centre is firm. Cover the handle of your skillet with foil before putting it in the oven if it has a plastic handle. Cut the frittata in half and serve with sour cream on top of each plate.

ADAPTABLE WITHOUT GLUTEN Make sure the prosciutto or Canadian bacon you use is gluten-free.

ADAPTABLE TO VEGETARIANS Remove the bacon/prosciutto from the recipe.

TIP Don't season the food with salt until after you've tasted it. The bacon/prosciutto will supply plenty of sodium on its own.

Try different cheese varieties and vegetable additions, such as Swiss cheese, zucchini, and sun-dried tomato.

pancakes with cinnamon rolls

This recipe makes eight 5-inch pancakes. Time to Prepare: 25 minutes 10 minutes to prepare

There is nothing more delightful on this planet than a warm cinnamon roll with cream cheese spilling down the sides.
It occurred to me one Sunday morning that pancakes, too, deserved that cinnamon–cream cheese bliss. Pancakes with crusty cinnamon craters were the end result. They resemble cinnamon rolls thanks to a generous spray of cream cheese icing.

FILLING WITH CINNAMON

4 tablespoons unsalted butter (12 stick), melted

SUPER CUTE RECIPES

14 cup light brown sugar + 2 teaspoons packed

12 teaspoons cinnamon powder

GLAZE WITH CREAM CHEESE

4 tablespoons unsalted butter (12 stick)

2 ounces room temperature cream cheese

34 cup sifted powdered sugar

12 teaspoon extract de vanille

PANCAKES

1 cup flour (all-purpose)

2 tblsp. baking powder

12 teaspoon sodium chloride

1 cup milk

1 lightly beaten big egg

1 tablespoon oil from canola

To make the cinnamon filling, combine the butter, brown sugar, and cinnamon in a medium mixing basin. Fill a quart-size hefty zip baggie halfway with the filling. Put something aside (see Tips).

Melt the butter in a small saucepan over low heat to make the glaze. Whisk in the cream cheese until it is completely smooth.

Turn off the heat in the pan. Set aside the powdered sugar and vanilla extract.

To make the pancake batter, whisk together the flour, baking powder, and salt in a medium mixing basin. Just until the batter is wet, whisk in the milk, egg, and oil (a few small lumps are fine).

Heat a big skillet or griddle over medium heat to make the pancakes. Using nonstick spray, coat the pan. To transfer the batter to the skillet, use an ice cream scoop or a 13 cup measuring cup. Spread the batter into a neat, even circle with the bottom of the scoop or cup (about 5 inches in diameter). Reduce the heat to a low setting. Using the cinnamon filling, snip the corner of the baggie and squeeze the filling into the open corner. Squeeze the cinnamon filling on top of the pancake batter in a swirl starting in the middle (just as you see in a regular cinnamon roll; see Tips). Cook the pancake for 3 to 4 minutes, or until bubbles emerge and burst on the top and the bottom is golden brown. Slide a thin spatula underneath the pancake and flip it over softly yet quickly. Cook for another 2 to 3 minutes until the opposite side is browned. When you turn the pancake onto a platter, you'll notice a crater-swirl of cinnamon generated by the cinnamon filling. Repeat with the nonstick spray and the remaining pancake batter and cinnamon filling, wiping off the pan with a paper towel. Serve the pancakes with a warm cream cheese glaze drizzled on top.

TIPS Before swirling the cinnamon filling, reopen the baggie and toss it well to include any butter that has separated. You want the mixture to thicken slightly—best it's if it resembles the squeezing texture of toothpaste, which will happen if you let it sit at room temperature for a few minutes (refrigerate it for a few minutes if you need to). If the filling hasn't hardened enough to produce a solid swirl, don't try to use it for the pancake swirl.

Pour the batter into the skillet, wait about a minute, and then swirl the cinnamon into the batter. This will allow the batter to set slightly before adding the swirl.

A FAST AND EASY TIP For this recipe, start with a boxed pancake mix.

If you're attempting to explain your indulgence in luscious cinnamon rolls, make this healthier by using half whole wheat flour and low-fat cream cheese, or skip the frosting entirely.

Chapter Twenty-one

Pancakes with pumpkin spice

Serves 4 to 6 people 15-minute prep time 6 to 8 minutes each pancake to cook

It's a fairly straightforward concept. When you combine pumpkin puree and spices with pancake batter, you'll get soft, moist, and fluffy pancakes that require little garnishing. When autumn arrives, I recommend stocking up on canned pumpkin puree. It can be difficult to come by in the middle of July, but you'll be craving these pumpkin pancakes all year.

2 1⁄2 cup flour (all-purpose)

1⁄4 cup light brown sugar, packed

1 tablespoon baking powder + 1 teaspoon baking soda

2 tablespoons cinnamon powder

1 teaspoon allspice powder

1 tblsp. salt

2 quarts milk

2/3 cup pumpkin puree, unsweetened

4 tablespoons unsalted butter (12 stick), melted

2 eggs, big

1 teaspoon essence of vanilla

For serving, combine butter and powdered sugar, as well as hot maple syrup.

Whisk together the flour, sugar, baking powder, cinnamon, allspice, and salt in a medium mixing basin.

Whisk together the milk, pumpkin, butter, eggs, and vanilla in a separate large mixing basin. Stir in the dry ingredients until barely mixed.

Over medium heat, preheat a large skillet or griddle. Using nonstick spray, coat the pan. To add the batter to the centre of the skillet, use an ice cream scoop (2 scoops) or a 12 cup measuring cup. Spread the batter into a neat, even circle with the bottom of the scoop or cup. Reduce the heat to medium-low and cook the pancake for 3 to 4 minutes, or until bubbles emerge and burst on top and the bottom is turning golden brown. Cook for a further 2 to 3 minutes on the opposite side until golden brown. Repeat with the remaining pancake batter and nonstick spray. Serve with butter and powdered sugar, as well as warm maple syrup.

TIP I prefer to heat the skillet to medium and then turn it down to medium-low after the pancakes start to cook. It gives the pancakes a head start in the cooking process, but you don't want to keep the heat that high for the entire cooking time or you'll get a tough crust.

To make pumpkin-pecan pancakes, add roasted pecans.

Add a cinnamon swirl filling and a cream cheese icing to turn these become Pumpkin–Cinnamon Roll Pancakes. For this variant, use the same swirling and topping directions as the Cinnamon Roll Pancakes recipe.

Chapter Twenty-two

Griddle cakes with bacon and corn

This recipe makes eight 4-inch griddle cakes. Time to Prepare: 25 minutes Time to prepare: 25 minutes

To be honest, we are typically a banana-pancake household. In the Recipe Girl household, a plain pancake is rarely served. Bananas are almost often chopped up and cooked right alongside the batter. Simply said, this is how we make pancakes around here. However, I was feeling a little crazy one weekend morning when I came up with this pancake recipe, and I surprised my family with a savoury pancake. It's a pancake with corn, bacon, and melted cheese on top, but no bananas. These have become a website favourite with extra bacon sprinkled on top and a heavy splash of maple syrup.

8 bacon slices, cut into 12-inch sections

13 cup sweet onion, coarsely chopped

1 cup flour (all-purpose)

2 tablespoons fresh chives, chopped

1 teaspoon powdered baking soda

12 teaspoon sodium chloride

cayenne pepper, 1/8 teaspoon

⅔ cup milk

1 big beaten egg

1 tablespoon vegetable or canola oil

1 cup corn kernels (frozen, canned, or fresh)

12 cup Monterey Jack cheese, shredded

For serving, warm maple syrup

Cook the bacon chunks in a medium skillet over medium-high heat until they begin to brown. Cook until the bacon is crisp and the onion is softened, then add the onion. Set aside a heaping tablespoon of the bacon mixture to decorate the griddle cakes.

Combine the flour, chives, baking powder, salt, and cayenne in a medium basin while the bacon is cooking. Just until moistened, stir in the milk, egg, and oil. Combine the leftover bacon mixture, corn, and cheese in a mixing bowl. It will be a

GRIDDLE CAKES WITH BACON AND CORN

thick mixture. If you want the griddle cakes to be thinner, thin out the mixture with a little additional milk.

Preheat a big skillet or griddle over medium heat. Using nonstick spray, coat the pan. Scoop a heaping 14 cup of batter onto the griddle and spread it out evenly using the bottom of the cup. Cook the griddle cake for 3 to 4 minutes per side, or until golden brown. Repeat with the remaining batter and nonstick spray.

Stack the griddle cakes and serve with a drizzle of the reserved bacon mixture and warm maple syrup on top.

ADAPTABLE TO VEGETARIANS Replace the bacon with veggie sausage.

TIP Cook your pancakes in the bacon fat from the skillet where you fried the bacon for a more indulgent option.

Chopped ham, green and red bell peppers, hot sauce, jalapeo cheese, and sausage are some other options for this delicious pancake.

fluffy, delicious pancakes

Serves 4 people Time to prepare: 10 minutes + rest time 4 minutes each pancake to cook

I've always been on the lookout for the ideal pancake. Good pancakes are light and fluffy. Thick and bubbling batter is ideal. On the griddle, the pancakes should bubble up a lot and keep their shape when piled with maple syrup drizzling down the edges. In this recipe, I believe I've perfected the fluffy pancake.

2 cups flour (all-purpose)

2 teaspoons white granulated sugar

2 tblsp. baking powder

1 teaspoon bicarbonate of soda

12 teaspoon sodium chloride

12 gallon buttermilk

½ cup milk

2 eggs, big

4 tablespoons salted butter (12 stick) melted

1 teaspoon essence of vanilla

For serving, warm maple syrup

Sift together the flour, sugar, baking powder, baking soda, and salt in a medium mixing basin.

Whisk together the buttermilk, milk, and eggs in a separate medium basin. Whisk in the melted butter and vanilla extract slowly.

Combine the wet and dry ingredients in a mixing bowl and stir gently with a fork. Only stir the batter until it is mostly incorporated. That's exactly what you want: a thick, lumpy batter. Allow 15 minutes for the batter to rest in the refrigerator.

Over medium heat, preheat a large skillet or griddle. Use a nonstick spray to coat it. To add the batter to the centre of the skillet, use an ice cream scoop (2 scoops) or a 12 cup measuring cup. Spread the batter into a neat, even circle with the bottom of the scoop or cup. It will be a thick batter. Cook the pancakes for 2 to 3 minutes, or until bubbles emerge on top and burst, and they are golden brown on the bottom. Cook for a further 1 to 2 minutes after flipping the pancakes until the other sides are golden brown. Repeat with the remaining batter and nonstick spray. Warm maple syrup is served on the side.

TIP Allowing the batter to rest in the refrigerator is essential. Resting the mixture allows the glutens in the flour to relax, resulting in more soft and fluffy pancakes, while keeping the batter cool prevents the baking powder and soda from activating too soon.

Chapter Twenty-three

Crunchy cinnamon crusted french toast

Approximately 6 slices 15-minute prep time Time to cook: 8 minutes

When I was little, I believe my mother prepared French toast every weekend. That's how I like to remember it, at least. I'm sure she kept things simple... It was only made with milk, eggs, and cinnamon, but that's what made it so delicious. My version is similarly basic, but with a cinnamon graham cracker crumb crust clinging to the custard-soaked bread.

34 gallon full milk (see Tips)

three huge eggs

2 tablespoons cinnamon powder, divided

12 tsp vanilla extract

12 graham crackers, broken into tiny crumbs with cinnamon

SUPER CUTE RECIPES

3 tblsp salted butter (divided)

6 sandwich bread slices (or thin-cut French bread)

For serving, warm maple syrup

Whisk together the milk, eggs, 1 teaspoon cinnamon, and vanilla in a medium, low, wide bowl. In a separate low wide bowl, combine the graham cracker crumbs and the remaining 1 teaspoon cinnamon.

Over medium heat, heat a large skillet or griddle. 1 tablespoon butter, melted and swirled about in the skillet to coat the bottom. 1 slice of bread should be dipped in the milk mixture and then into the crumbs to coat both sides. In the skillet, place the bread. Rep with as many slices as the skillet will hold. Cook for 3 to 4 minutes, or until the bread is brown and toasted on the bottom. Cook for a further 2 to 3 minutes on the opposite side until golden brown. Continue with the remaining butter, bread slices, and dipping sauces. Warm maple syrup on top.

TIPS If you like, half-and-half can be used instead of whole milk. It'll merely add to the decadence of your French toast. On the other hand, nonfat milk should be avoided because it results in soggy French toast.

Use normal graham crackers and add an additional 12 tsp cinnamon to the crushed crumbs if you only have regular graham crackers in your pantry.

CRUNCHY CINNAMON CRUSTED FRENCH TOAST

This recipe, made using Hawaiian egg bread or challah, is a family favourite. Both types of bread should be available in the bread aisle or bakery of your local supermarket.

Add 14 cup unsweetened pumpkin puree, 1 tablespoon granulated white sugar, and 14 teaspoon ground nutmeg to your milk mixture to make Pumpkin French Toast. With those extra ingredients, you'll be able to dip 8 slices of bread into the custard.

Chapter Twenty-four

Kahla–brown sugar bananas on challah french toast

Serves 4 people 20-minute prep time Time to prepare: 25 minutes

My husband and I once spent a romantic weekend in Montecito, a charming tiny town near Santa Barbara. We ate local fish and homemade ice cream, looked for Oprah (a local resident) but couldn't find her, and then discovered "Jeannine's," the most incredible brunch spot. I'm glad the pastries and desserts were in a glass case because I might have helped myself. My husband selected their Kahla French Toast with Sautéed Bananas, popularly known as Heaven on a Plate, which was a thing of beauty with freshly sliced strawberries and huge juicy blueberries. This recipe is inspired by Jeannine's delicious French toast.

BANANAS

SUPER CUTE RECIPES

8 tablespoons salted butter (1 stick)

34 cup light brown sugar, packed

3 big sliced bananas

14 cup of Kahla

TOAST FRENCH

a dozen big eggs

12 gallon whole milk

12 teaspoon extract de vanille

12 teaspoon cinnamon powder

1/8 teaspoon nutmeg powder

34 pound challah loaf, cut into 1-inch thick slices (8 slices)

Melt the butter in a medium skillet over medium heat to prepare the bananas. Combine the brown sugar and bananas in a mixing bowl. Cook the bananas for 4 to 5 minutes, stirring frequently, until the mixture thickens. Cook for an additional 2 to 3 minutes, or until the bananas are mushy and the sauce has thickened to a syrup consistency. Take the skillet from the heat, cover it, and set it aside.

To make the French toast, mix together the eggs, milk, vanilla, cinnamon, and nutmeg in a low, wide bowl. Preheat a medium-sized skillet over medium heat. Use a nonstick spray

KAHLA–BROWN SUGAR BANANAS ON CHALLAH FRENCH NO.1

to coat it. 1 slice of bread should be dipped in the egg mixture on both sides. In the skillet, place the bread. Rep with as many slices as the skillet will hold. Cook for 3 to 4 minutes, or until the bread is golden brown on the bottom. Cook for an additional 2 to 3 minutes on the other side, or until golden brown on both sides. Repeat with the remaining bread and nonstick spray. Serve the French toast with a scoop of the bananas that were set aside.

ADAPTABLE WITHOUT GLUTEN In place of the Challah, use your favourite gluten-free bread.

TIPS This French toast does not require the use of any syrup. The bananas serve as a luscious and delicious topping.

It's fine to leave the alcohol out of the sauce if you don't want to use it in the dish. Simply replace the Kahla with a tablespoon of maple syrup.

In addition, the banana sauce is delicious as an ice cream topping.

Instead, serve with a peach–brown sugar topping. Replace the bananas with peeled and sliced peaches, and the Kahla with 1 tablespoon vanilla extract.

Chapter Twenty-five

Waffles with apple bacon and cider syrup

Approximately 6 servings Time to Prepare: 25 minutes 3 to 5 minutes per waffle to cook

If I could, I'd put bacon in everything. That smokey flavour and mild crunch goes well with just about everything. You can skip the process of serving bacon on the side with these waffles. You simply put the bacon pieces into the waffle batter and savour bacon in every mouthful; it also goes well with the apple, which is another hidden ingredient in these waffles. Breakfast is complete with the addition of a sweet cider syrup.

SYRUP OF CIDER

12 cup white granulated sugar

cornstarch, 1 tablespoon

a quarter teaspoon of pumpkin pie spice

1 cup apple cider, unsweetened

1 tablespoon lemon juice, freshly squeezed

2 tablespoons butter, salted

WAFFLES

12 cup flour (all-purpose)

2 teaspoons white granulated sugar

12 teaspoon bicarbonate of soda

12 teaspoon sodium chloride

a quarter-cup of buttermilk

¾ cup milk

8 tablespoons salted butter (1 stick) melted

three huge eggs

1 medium peeled, cored, and shredded apple (see Tips)

8 cooked and crumbled bacon slices

To make the cider syrup, combine the sugar, cornstarch, and pumpkin pie spice in a medium pot. Combine the cider and lemon juice in a mixing bowl. Bring the mixture to a boil over medium heat, stirring frequently. Reduce the heat to low and keep the mixture simmering until it thickens. Remove the pan

WAFFLES WITH APPLE BACON AND CIDER SYRUP

from the heat and butter it. Stir until the butter has melted and the syrup is fully mixed.

Preheat your waffle iron as directed by the manufacturer.

To make the waffles, whisk together the flour, sugar, baking soda, and salt in a medium mixing basin. Combine the buttermilk, milk, butter, and eggs in a separate large mixing basin. Stir in the dry ingredients until barely mixed. Combine the apple and bacon in a mixing bowl.

Apply nonstick spray to the preheated waffle iron. Fill your waffle iron halfway with batter and close the lid. Depending on the sort of waffle iron you have, the waffles should take 3 to 5 minutes to cook. Rep with the rest of the batter. Waffles should be served with warm cider syrup.

TIPS Granny Smith, Braeburn, and Jonathon apples are the best for pancakes.

2 to 3 days before serving, make the cider syrup. Keep it covered and refrigerated until you're ready to serve it.

Waffles can be made ahead of time and frozen. To reheat them, place them in the toaster.

Try substituting turkey bacon for normal bacon. Extra bacon can be fried and crumbled on top of individual portions.

maple bacon roasted in the oven

Makes: 12 bacon strips Time to Prepare: 10 minutes 18 minutes to prepare

It changed my life forever the first time I baked bacon in the oven. It's no longer necessary to cram large strips of bacon into a round pan. No more splattering oil all over my cooktop from a large skillet, and no more burning bacon in the pan because I'm too preoccupied with other things. This bacon is cooked to perfection, crispy on the outside and full of flavour.

a dozen bacon slices (see Tips)

2 tsp. maple syrup

12 teaspoon mustard (Dijon) black pepper, freshly ground

Preheat the oven to 400 degrees Fahrenheit. Place a rack on top of a rimmed baking sheet with enough foil to come up and over the sides. Using nonstick spray, coat the rack.

On the rack, arrange the bacon strips. Bake for 15 minutes, or until the bacon begins to colour.

Prepare the maple glaze while the bacon is baking. Whisk together the syrup and mustard in a medium shallow bowl until smooth.

When the bacon has finished cooking for 15 minutes, carefully remove the skillet from the oven and brush the maple glaze over the bacon slices. Add the pepper to the top. Return the pan to the oven for another 3 minutes, or until the bacon is crisp and brown. Serve immediately after draining the fat from the bottom of the bacon strips on a paper towel–lined plate.

ADAPTABLE WITHOUT GLUTEN Make sure the bacon, Dijon mustard, and maple syrup you use are gluten-free.

TIP Depending on the thickness of the bacon you're using, the timing may vary slightly. The directions are for standard sliced bacon. Cooking thick-sliced bacon may take a little longer.

To make a spicy sweet dessert, replace the pepper with a sprinkling of cinnamon.

Instead of maple syrup, use honey to make honey-glazed bacon.

Chapter Twenty-six

Breakfast potatoes by Susie

Serves 12 people Time to prepare: 35 minutes plus cooling time 45 minutes to prepare

Susie, my younger sister, has always had the most delicious recipes. I used to go see my older sister in college and spend hours pouring through her cookbooks and recipe collections, jotting down dishes I wanted to try out someday. This recipe is based on one that I copied down many years ago. It has since become our family's go-to breakfast potato recipe to serve alongside egg casseroles or baked ham at huge holiday brunch gatherings. It's easy to make and excellent.

5 to 6 medium russet or Yukon gold potatoes, washed and split in half

4 tablespoons salted butter (12 stick)

12 cup onion, finely chopped

12 cup red bell pepper, finely chopped

1 tablespoon flour (all-purpose)

12 c. chicken stock

½ cup milk

sour cream, 2 cups

1 cup sharp cheddar cheese, shredded

1 tablespoon salt

14 teaspoon pepper, freshly ground

1 cup cornflakes, crushed

Preheat the oven to 350 degrees Fahrenheit. Using nonstick spray, coat a 9 x 13-inch pan.

Bring a big saucepan of water to a rolling boil. Boil for 20 minutes with the potatoes (skin on). Drain the water and allow the potatoes to cool until they are safe to handle (about 20 minutes). Remove the skin and throw it away. Grate the potatoes into the pan that has been prepared.

Melt the butter in a medium saucepan over medium heat. Cook for 3 to 4 minutes, until the onion and bell pepper are softened and gently browned. Incorporate the flour. Slowly pour in the chicken broth, followed by the milk. Bring the mixture to a boil, stirring constantly, until the sauce has thickened somewhat. Stir in the sour cream, cheese, salt, and pepper until the cheese is completely melted. Over the potatoes, pour the sauce. On top, sprinkle the crushed cornflakes.

Bake for 45 to 60 minutes, or until the potatoes are heated, bubbling, and turning golden brown.

ADAPTABLE WITHOUT GLUTEN Use potato starch or cornstarch instead of all-purpose flour as a thickening. Make sure the chicken broth and cornflakes you use are gluten-free.

ADAPTABLE TO VEGETARIANS In place of chicken broth, use vegetarian broth.

TIP Reduced-fat sour cream works perfectly in this recipe. Low-fat cheese, on the other hand, does not melt well and should be avoided.

A FAST AND EASY TIP Instead of fresh potatoes, use one 2-pound box of defrosted frozen hash brown potatoes.

Add chopped green bell peppers to make this a festive Christmas brunch meal.

Chapter Twenty-seven

Almond-cranberry granola

4 cup serving 20-minute prep time Time to prepare: 25 minutes

"Why would you make granola when you can just purchase it at the store?" my husband asked when I informed him I was working on a granola recipe for the cookbook. Mr. Recipe Husband, I'll tell you why: It's extremely simple to make, I know exactly what I'm putting in it, and it's absolutely wonderful! And having a good stash of handmade granola on hand makes me happy because I eat a sprinkle of granola on my Greek yoghurt virtually every day of my life. So there.

2 cups oats, old-fashioned

1 cup unsalted whole almonds, coarsely chopped

Optional: 12 cup unsweetened coconut flakes

13 cup oat bran, flaxseed powder, or wheat germ

12 teaspoon cinnamon powder

1 tablespoon salt

1 pound honey

14 cup canola or vegetable oil

14 cup orange juice, freshly squeezed

2 tbsp. light brown sugar, packed

12 teaspoon extract de vanille

12 cup cranberries, dried

Preheat the oven to 325 degrees Fahrenheit. Using nonstick spray, coat a rimmed baking sheet.

Toss the oats, almonds, coconut flakes, oat bran, cinnamon, and salt together in a large mixing dish.

Whisk together the honey, oil, orange juice, sugar, and vanilla in a medium mixing basin. Stir in the wet ingredients until well combined.

Pour the mixture onto the baking sheet that has been prepared. Bake for 15 minutes before stirring. Bake for another 5–10 minutes, or until the oats are golden brown (keep an eye on the granola at this point to make sure it doesn't brown too much). Remove the granola from the oven, toss in the dried cranberries, and set aside to cool.

Scoop the granola into a closed container once it has cooled fully. It will keep for up to 2 weeks.

ADAPTABLE WITHOUT GLUTEN Make sure the oats and dried cranberries you use are gluten-free. Instead of wheat germ, use ground flax or gluten-free oat bran.

TIP While baking, the oats will remain mushy, but once cooled, they will crisp up.

IDEA FOR GIFT For a delightful, homemade gift, spoon the granola into small plastic gift bags and tie on colourful ribbons and labels.

Chapter Twenty-eight

Applesauce with maple and cinnamon

3 cup serving Time to Prepare: 25 minutes 45 minutes to prepare

Where I live in Southern California, the fall season is practically non-existent. Unfortunately, we miss the changing colours of the leaves and the coolness that signals the start of a new season. We continue to get 75-degree days long into November, when the leaves all fall off the trees at once, dead rather than multicoloured. Every September, we go apple picking in the local mountains, where we can wear our fleece coats and do some serious apple picking. In my house, those apples end up as applesauce, sweetened with maple syrup and seasoned with cinnamon.

10 apples, medium (see Tips)

1 cup of water

14 cup maple syrup, pure (see Tips)

1 teaspoon lemon juice, freshly squeezed

12 teaspoon cinnamon powder

a quarter teaspoon allspice

All of the apples should be cored and peeled before being chopped into 1-inch chunks and placed in a medium pot. Stir in the remaining ingredients in the pan. Heat the mixture over medium-high heat, checking underneath the apples to see if the liquid has come to a boil. Reduce the heat to the lowest setting possible and stir once more. Cover the pan and cook for 45 to 1 hour, stirring every 15 minutes, until the apples soften and break apart.

Remove the skillet from the heat and mash the apples with a fork or a potato masher until they achieve the desired applesauce consistency. Serve warm, or keep refrigerated and serve cold later.

TIPS Using a few different apple kinds gives the applesauce a nice flavour. McIntosh, Golden Delicious, Cortland, Empire, Fuji, Spartan, and Winesap are some of my favourites.

The majority of pancake syrup offered is not genuine maple syrup. These syrups are manufactured primarily of cane sugar or corn syrup, with a minor amount of maple syrup added for flavour. Pure maple syrup is ideal for cooking and baking since it has a stronger maple flavour. On the label, look for Grade A or B.

Keep the applesauce in a closed container in the refrigerator for up to 2 weeks.

The applesauce produced by this recipe is chunky. If you like pureed applesauce, let the apples cool before transferring them to a food processor.

Chapter Twenty-nine

Blueberry-oatmeal breakfast bars

Approximately 12 bars 20-minute prep time Time to prepare: 20 minutes

The ability to have breakfast in one's hand and walk out the door appeals to many people in today's fast-paced environment of apparently nonstop hectic family activities. Breakfast on the run need not be unhealthy. These whole wheat bars with dried blueberries, pecans, and oats are mildly sweetened. They fill your stomach with a pleasant little treat in the morning without putting you on a sugar high. It's a pleasant way to begin the day.

34 cup flour (whole wheat)

34 cup flour (all-purpose)

34 cup quick-cooking or old-fashioned oats

1 teaspoon cinnamon powder

12 teaspoon bicarbonate of soda

a quarter teaspoon of salt

1 pound honey

13 cup applesauce, unsweetened

13 gallon nonfat milk

4 tablespoons salted butter (12 stick) melted

1 egg, big

2 tbsp. light brown sugar, packed

1 teaspoon essence of vanilla

1 cup blueberries, dry

12 cup pecans, roughly chopped

Preheat the oven to 350 degrees Fahrenheit. Nonstick spray a 9-inch square pan or a 7-inch 11-inch pan.

Combine the flours, oats, cinnamon, baking soda, and salt in a medium mixing basin. Whisk together the honey, applesauce, milk, butter, egg, sugar, and vanilla in a separate medium basin. Stir in the remaining dry ingredients. Stir in the blueberries and pecans until well mixed (see Tips).

Scrape the batter into the pan and smooth the top to make it even. Bake for 20–22 minutes, or until a toothpick inserted in the middle comes out clean. Serve by cutting into bars.

TIPS Avoid overmixing the batter, since this will result in a harsher, denser texture.

When maintained in a sealed container, these bars will last 2 to 3 days at room temperature. Alternatively, freeze bars for up to a month in individual zip baggies, then defrost as needed for a quick breakfast.

Replace the blueberries with another dried fruit and nut combination, such as apricot/almond, cherry/almond, or apple/walnut.

WEB VEGETARIAN FAVORITE (or adaptable) GRAIN-FREE (or adaptable) NON-DAIRY (or adaptable)

Soup with tomato, basil, and garlic-cheese croutons

Serves 4 to 6 people Time to prepare: 40 minutes plus cooling time 1 hour to prepare

The greatest way to enjoy tomato soup is with a grilled cheese sandwich for dipping. When I was younger, I used to make my tomato soup with cubes of bread and chunks of cheddar cheese to speed up the sandwich-making process. Every bite would include a slice of bread and melting cheese strands. It worked perfectly. Instead of croutons, my grown-up tomato soup has homemade garlic-cheese croutons, which appears to be the ideal option for satisfying the grilled cheese and tomato soup craving.

SUPER CUTE RECIPES

CROUTONS

4 cups stale French bread, cubed

4 tablespoons salted butter (12 stick) melted

1 teaspoon powdered garlic

12 teaspoon seasoning (Italian)

14 cup Parmesan cheese, freshly grated

SOUP

1 tablespoon butter (salted)

1 sliced tiny onion (about 1 cup)

1 peeled and coarsely chopped tiny carrot

1 celery stalk, finely chopped

1 teaspoon garlic, minced

balsamic vinegar, 1 tbsp

2 tblsp flour (all-purpose)

1 San Marzano tomato can (28 ounces) (see Tips)

1 quart vegetable stock

1 tablespoon basil, finely chopped

12 teaspoon white granulated sugar

12 teaspoon salt (kosher)

cayenne pepper, 1/8 teaspoon

1 to 2 cups one percent milk

Preheat the oven to 350 degrees Fahrenheit for the croutons. Toss the bread pieces, butter, garlic powder, and Italian seasoning in a medium mixing basin. Place the bread on a rimmed baking sheet and spread it out. Cheese should be sprinkled on top. 15 minutes in the oven Let cool.

Melt the butter in a medium skillet over medium heat to make the soup. Combine the onion, carrot, and celery in a bowl. Cook, stirring occasionally, for 4 to 5 minutes, or until the veggies are softened. Cook for 1 minute after adding the garlic. Add the vinegar, whisk to combine the veggies, and then add the flour. Stir once more. Toss in the tomatoes and the broth. Bring the mixture to a boil by increasing the heat to high. Reduce the heat to low and cover the skillet. 30 minutes on low heat Remove the pan from the heat and add the basil, sugar, salt, and cayenne pepper. Allow 15 minutes for cooling.

Fill a food processor or blender halfway with the mixture. Blend until completely smooth. In a big saucepan, pour the pureed soup. Rep with the rest of the mixture. 12 cup milk should be added at this point. Depending on how thin you want your soup, add up to 12 cup more. Warm the soup over medium heat until it is thoroughly cooked. Serve the soup in warmed cups with the croutons on top (see Tips).

ADAPTABLE WITHOUT GLUTEN Use gluten-free bread to make the croutons. In place of all-purpose flour, thicken the soup with a gluten-free flour mix or potato starch.

TIPS San Marzano tomatoes are a plum tomato cultivar that many consider to make the tastiest sauces. Marzanos in cans are available at most well-stocked supermarket stores. If you can't get fresh Italian plum tomatoes, tinned Italian plum tomatoes will suffice.

Any leftover croutons can be stored in an airtight jar for up to 2 weeks. They're also delicious in salads.

Whipping cream, rather than milk, can be used to make this soup creamier.

Serve this soup with grilled cheese sandwich half instead of croutons if you don't want to make the croutons.

Chapter Thirty

Beef and lentil soup in a slow cooker

Serves 4 people Time to Prepare: 25 minutes Time to prepare: 8 hours

It's a little surprising that I have more than one slow cooker dish in this book. Slow cooker meals have never been my favourite. I've tried a lot of them, but only a few make it into my "recipes to try again" folder. Still, I'm looking for fantastic slow cooker recipes! I'm short on time and need a soup that will nourish my hubby for a few days. Soups like this one, which contains beef, lentils, and a variety of vegetables, are filling for lunch and robust enough for dinner, especially when served with a good piece of Italian bread to mop up the broth. This is one of those dishes that you'll want to make again and again.

2 tblsp. extra virgin olive oil, divided

1 pound boneless chuck roast, sliced into 12 inch chunks

1⁄3 cup red wine, dry (see Tips)

1 cup celery, chopped

1 cup leek, thinly sliced (only white and light green bits)

1 cup peeled and thinly sliced carrots

1 teaspoon garlic, minced

3 quarts beef stock

3 quarts of water

1 small diced tomato (14.5-ounce can)

1 cup lentils, dried

1 bay leaf

3 cups spinach, trimmed and discarding stems

1 tablespoon oregano, chopped

To taste, season with salt and freshly ground black pepper.

In a large skillet, heat 1 tablespoon of olive oil over medium heat. Cook, tossing frequently, until the beef is browned on all sides, about 5 to 6 minutes. Deglaze the skillet with wine, scraping up any browned bits from the bottom. Fill your slow cooker with the meat and liquids.

With a paper towel, wipe clean the skillet and heat the remaining 1 tablespoon of oil over medium heat. Cook, stirring

BEEF AND LENTIL SOUP IN A SLOW COOKER

occasionally, until the celery, leek, and carrot have softened, about 4 to 5 minutes. Cook for a further minute after adding the garlic. Fill the slow cooker with the vegetable mixture. In a slow cooker, combine the broth, water, tomatoes, lentils, and bay leaf. Cook on low for 7 to 8 hours, or high for 312 to 4 hours, covered. Remove the bay leaf and toss in the spinach and oregano when ready to serve the soup. Taste to determine if any salt or freshly ground black pepper is needed.

ADAPTABLE WITHOUT GLUTEN Make sure the beef broth you're using is gluten-free.

TIPS When using red wine in cooking, choose a wine that you enjoy drinking. This recipe benefits from Cabernet Sauvignon.

If you don't have a slow cooker, use a Dutch oven to make the soup. Follow the same directions and cook on low heat for 35 to 45 minutes, or until the lentils are cooked.

MAKE-AHEAD SUGGESTIONS The night before, prepare everything and place it in your slow cooker's pot (leaving out the lentils). Simply add the lentils the next day and continue the slow-cooking process as directed.

Replace the leeks with onions.

Replace the oregano with fresh thyme or rosemary to change the flavour of the soup. Alternatively, combine herbs.

Another fantastic addition to this soup is Swiss chard. Remove the ribs and finely slice the leaves. Remove the spinach and add it towards the end of the soup.

Chapter Thirty-one

Clam chowder from New England

Approximately 6 servings 20-minute prep time Time to prepare: 20 minutes

Haddad's Ocean Café in Brant Rock, Massachusetts, serves the best clam chowder (chowdah). The key, according to owner Chuck Haddad, is a lot of buttah! I can only add so much butter to my recipe before I start worrying about how tight my jeans will fit the next day. This is my family's special clam chowder recipe, which we've been eating and enjoying for many years. I've tweaked our original recipe to make it worthy of a cookbook and comparable to (or, dare I say, better than) Haddad's chowder.

SOUP

1 tablespoon butter (salted)

1 cup onion, chopped

1 cup celery, chopped

2 cups red potato, diced and unpeeled

1 clam juice bottle (8 oz.)

2 6-ounce clam cans (with juice)

12 teaspoon sodium chloride

SAUCE WHITE

8 tablespoons salted butter (1 stick)

12 cup flour (all-purpose)

2 c. cream of tartar

2 quarts of whole milk

2 bay leaves (optional)

12 tbsp fresh thyme, chopped

1 tablespoon salt

1/8 teaspoon black pepper, freshly ground

ADDITIVES (OPTIONAL)

6 cooked and crumbled bacon slices (see Tips)

Vinegar of red wine

Melt the butter in a large pot over medium heat to make the soup. Cook, stirring occasionally, until the onion and celery

CLAM CHOWDER FROM NEW ENGLAND

soften, about 3 to 4 minutes. Combine the potato, bottled clam juice, and the clam liquid from the cans. Just cover the vegetables with adequate water. Add the salt and mix well. Bring the liquid to a moderate simmer and continue to cook until the potatoes are cooked, about 8 to 10 minutes.

Prepare the white sauce while the potatoes are cooking. Melt the butter in a separate big saucepan over medium heat. In a mixing bowl, combine the flour and butter. Whisk in the half-and-half and milk slowly. Toss in the bay leaves. Bring to a boil over medium-high heat, whisking constantly until slightly thickened, 3 to 5 minutes.

Toss the remaining soup with the white sauce. Simmer the clams, thyme, salt, and pepper over low heat. Simmer for 3 to 4 minutes, or until the soup is well heated. If desired, serve the soup in bowls with crumbled bacon and a drizzle of red wine vinegar.

ADAPTABLE WITHOUT GLUTEN In place of all-purpose flour, use 14 cup cornstarch, tapioca starch, or potato starch. Before adding it to the soup, mix it with a little cream. Use a gluten-free bacon brand that is well-known.

TIPS If you want, use 1 cup fresh clams instead of canned clams. You'll need another 12 cup of clam juice.

Cook your bacon in the oven for simple cleanup. Preheat the oven to 400 degrees Fahrenheit. Place a rack on top of a big, rimmed baking sheet lined with foil. Using nonstick spray, coat the rack. On the rack, arrange the bacon strips. Bake for 15 to 20 minutes, or until crisp. The length of time depends on how thick your bacon is.

Instead of cream and whole milk, use 2 cups whole milk and 2 cups nonfat milk to lighten up this soup. Your soup won't be quite as creamy and thick, but the flavour will be just as delicious.

Serve the soup in sourdough bowls hollowed out of little loaves of sourdough bread. Soup eaters can rip the dish apart and consume the bread as well!

Chapter Thirty-two

Vegetable soup from Italy

Approximately 8 servings 30 minute prep time Time to prepare: 25 minutes

I enjoy spaghetti, Mexican food, and desserts in particular. But every now and then, my body need some detox time. A substantial, healthful soup is ideal for such occasions. It has to be a soup with a lot of veggies and beans, maybe even a little potato, all combined in a rich and tasty broth. This veggie soup works wonders. It's full and deliciously cleansing. It's even nicer if you have a good hunk of crusty bread on hand to soak up the leftover liquid.

1 tablespoon extra virgin olive oil

12 big sliced onion

2 large leeks, thinly cut (white and light green sections), rinsed

4 minced medium garlic cloves

SUPER CUTE RECIPES

2 cups zucchini, chopped (2 medium)

2 cups carrots, chopped (3 medium)

2 cups finely sliced cabbage (14 head)

3 low-sodium chicken broth 14.5-ounce cans

2 small diced tomatoes (14.5 oz.)

1 washed and drained 15-ounce can of white beans

1 giant peeled and chopped potato (about 112 cups)

3 cups kale or Swiss chard, finely sliced (ribs removed)

1 cup corn kernels (fresh or frozen)

1 tablespoon oregano or basil, finely chopped

1 tblsp. salt

12 teaspoon black pepper, freshly ground

1 cup Parmesan cheese, freshly grated

Heat the olive oil in a big saucepan over medium heat. Cook, stirring occasionally, until the onion and leeks are softened, 3 to 4 minutes. Cook for a further minute after adding the garlic. Cook, stirring frequently, until the zucchini, carrot, and cabbage are slightly softened, 3 to 4 minutes. Combine the broth, tomatoes, beans, and potato in a mixing bowl. Bring the mixture to a boil, then reduce to a low heat and cook for 7 to 10 minutes, or until the potatoes are soft. Add the kale, corn, oregano, salt, and pepper to taste. Cook for 3 to 4 minutes, or until the kale is wilted and tender. To serve, ladle the soup into bowls and top with cheese.

ADAPTABLE WITHOUT GLUTEN Make sure the broth and beans you use are gluten-free.

TIP Preparing dinner is made easier by chopping veggies early in the day. Simply chop everything (except the potatoes) and store in covered containers in the fridge until ready to use!

To give the soup extra depth of flavour, add 12 cup Marsala wine, or a tablespoon of Marsala to individual servings, if preferred.

Red cabbage also works well in this soup and gives a lovely colour.

Add extra of your favourite vegetables to this soup, or make your own blend. Suggested vegetables include green beans, winter squash, and yellow squash.

Chapter Thirty-three

Soup with butternut squash, pancetta, and crispy sage

Serves 4 people 30 minute prep time 35 minutes to prepare

I'm pretty sure I could live entirely on butternut squash. For breakfast, I'd joyfully mash roasted squash into my porridge (well, not really, but for the sake of the story...), lunch would be roasted butternut squash with sage and garlic and goat cheese, and dinner would be butternut squash soup. I'm quite sure my family wouldn't let me dump my butternut squash infatuation on them, but when I do have a weekend to myself, it's all about butternut squash. My favourite soup recipe in the book is this one. The soup is gently sweet, and the crisp of pancetta and sage sprinkled on top is just right.

SOUP

1 tablespoon extra virgin olive oil

12 cup shallots, sliced

1 teaspoon garlic, minced

14 cup white wine, dry

2 low-sodium chicken broth 14-ounce cans

8 cups butternut squash, diced (about 3 pounds)

1 teaspoon maple sugar

To taste, season with salt and freshly ground black pepper.

TOPPINGS

4 ounces chopped pancetta

14 cup sage, julienned (see Tips)

To make the soup, heat the olive oil in a big, deep skillet over medium heat. Cook, stirring occasionally, until the shallot is gently caramelised and softened, 3 to 5 minutes. Cook for a further minute after adding the garlic. Deglaze the skillet with wine, scraping up any browned bits from the bottom. Stir in the squash after adding the broth. Bring to a boil, then lower to a low heat and cook for 20 to 30 minutes, or until the squash is cooked (see Tips). Remove the skillet from the heat and set aside for 15 minutes to cool.

Heat a medium skillet over medium heat for the toppings. Cook and toss the pancetta until it is browned and crispy, about 4 to 5 minutes. When the pancetta is crisp, add the sage and toss for a further minute, or until the sage is crispy.

SOUP WITH BUTTERNUT SQUASH, PANCETTA, AND CRISPY...

Transfer the pancetta and sage to a paper towel–lined dish using a slotted spoon. Allow it to cool and drain until the soup is ready to be served.

Fill a food processor or blender halfway with cooked squash and broth. Blend until completely smooth. In a big saucepan, pour the pureed soup. Continue with the rest of the squash and broth. Season with salt and pepper to taste after adding the maple syrup. Heat the soup over medium heat for 4 to 5 minutes, or until well heated. Serve the soup in cups or bowls with pancetta and crispy sage on top.

ADAPTABLE WITHOUT GLUTEN Make sure to use gluten-free brands of broth, maple syrup, and pancetta.

VEGETARIAN-ADAPTABLE Replace the chicken broth with vegetable broth and omit the pancetta.

TIPS Tender squash is defined as squash that can be pierced with a fork without exerting too much pressure. It should be soft without being mushy.

To julienne the sage, stack several leaves on top of one another. Cut the sage lengthwise with a sharp knife to create long, thin strips of fresh sage.

Leave out the maple syrup if you don't want a somewhat sweet soup. Alternatively, taste the soup as it is and gradually add a teaspoon of maple syrup until you get the desired sweetness.

soup with roasted carrots and sweet potatoes

Approximately 6 servings 30 minute prep time 1 hour and 10 minutes to prepare

Carrots have a reputation for being a bland vegetable. They're dipped in Ranch dressing to make them taste better, added to salads for colour, and taken from vegetable platters by default. However, roasting these earthy orange things in the oven with a sprinkle of olive oil transforms them into sweet, slightly irresistible vegetables. The tastes of roasted carrots and baked sweet potato mix to form a filling and nutritious soup. Even carrot sceptics would concur.

6 big carrots (about 1 pound), cut and peeled

12 tablespoons extra virgin olive oil

1 teaspoon kosher salt plus additional salt to taste

14 teaspoon black pepper, freshly ground + more to taste

1 large orange-fleshed sweet potato (approximately 1 pound), split in half, poked with a fork, and wrapped in foil in each half

2 tablespoons butter, salted

34 cup finely sliced onion (12 medium)

1 teaspoon garlic, minced (about 1 large clove)

3 cups veggie broth + more liquid as needed (see Tips)

SOUP WITH BUTTERNUT SQUASH, PANCETTA, AND CRISPY...

12 tbsp fresh thyme, chopped

14 teaspoon cumin powder

Optional lemon wedges for serving

Preheat the oven to 375 degrees Fahrenheit. Using nonstick spray, coat a rimmed baking sheet.

Carrots should be cut into 3-inch slices. Any larger pieces should be cut vertically to make them more uniform in size. Toss the carrots with the olive oil in the pan that has been prepared. 1 teaspoon salt and 14 teaspoon pepper, to taste Place the potatoes wrapped in foil on the baking sheet. Bake the carrots for 1 hour, stirring every 20 minutes (see Tips).

Melt the butter in a big, deep skillet over medium heat. Cook, stirring occasionally, until the onion is cooked and golden brown, about 4 to 5 minutes. Cook for an additional 1 minute, stirring constantly. Add the thyme and the broth. Remove from the heat and mix well.

In a food processor, combine half of the carrots, one potato half, and half of the broth mixture. Blend until completely smooth. In a big saucepan, pour the pureed soup. Replace the carrots, potato half, and broth as needed. Add the cumin and season with salt and pepper to taste. 3 to 5 minutes over medium heat, cook the soup until it is thoroughly heated. If desired, serve soup in dishes with lemon wedges for squeezing.

ADAPTABLE WITHOUT GLUTEN Make sure the broth you're using is gluten-free.

ADAPTABLE DAIRY-FREE To sauté the onions, substitute olive oil for butter.

TIPS If your soup appears to be overly thick, add more broth.

Watch out for your carrots. Remove the carrots from the oven before they get tender and lightly browned, and continue to roast the potatoes for the remaining time.

This soup can be made 1 to 2 days ahead of time and then reheated before serving. Because the flavours have a chance to deepen while sitting, leftovers are almost better than eating the same day.

Stir in half-and-half or whipping cream to make this a creamy soup. To make the soup sweeter, add a small amount of honey.

Chapter Thirty-four

Soup with roasted cherry tomatoes with macaroni and cheese

Serves 4 people 30 minute prep time 35 minutes to prepare

Right? I think we can all agree that macaroni and cheese is the ideal comfort dish. It's thick, velvety, cheesy, ooey, gooey, and ridiculously rich. Eating macaroni and cheese brings consolation in the sense that it satisfies one's desire to consume something so delicious. In this recipe, macaroni is used in a creamy cheese soup that is finished with delicately roasted tomatoes. Doesn't it seem like some nice comfort food right there?

TOMATOES

12 cherry tomatoes, half-cut (see Tips)

1 tablespoon extra virgin olive oil

freshly ground black pepper and salt

SOUP

2 tablespoons butter, salted

2 teaspoons garlic, minced (about 3 cloves)

2 tblsp flour (all-purpose)

6 c. vegetable stock

1 bay leaf

1 cup elbow macaroni, dry

1 quart heavy cream

1 tablespoon mustard (Dijon)

1 tbsp. Worcestershire

12 teaspoon Tabasco pepper sauce

12 teaspoon freshly ground white pepper

8 oz. extra-sharp cheddar cheese, shredded

Preheat the oven to 425°F for roasting the tomatoes. Place the tomatoes on a rimmed baking sheet, cut side up. Season with salt and pepper and drizzle with olive oil. 12 minutes to roast the tomatoes Remove them from the oven and set them aside to cool while you finish the soup.

Melt the butter in a large pot over medium heat to make the soup. Cook, stirring constantly, until the garlic is mellow and

SOUP WITH ROASTED CHERRY TOMATOES WITH MACARONI...

aromatic, about 1 minute. Incorporate the flour. Whisk in the veggie broth slowly, then add the bay leaf. Bring the broth to a boil by increasing the heat to high. Boil for about 8 minutes, or until the macaroni is almost tender. Remove and discard the bay leaf. Add the cream, mustard, Worcestershire sauce, Tabasco sauce, and pepper and stir to combine. Continue to whisk in the cheese until it is totally melted. Return the soup to a boil for 2 minutes, stirring occasionally, before turning off the heat. Serve the soup in serving bowls with the roasted tomatoes on top.

TIPS For this recipe, smaller cherry or pear tomatoes work best. Larger cherry tomatoes may require a slightly longer roasting time or cutting into fourths.

When leftovers are refrigerated, the pasta has more time to soak up the liquid in the soup, resulting in a beautifully creamy macaroni and cheese.

The beautiful thing about macaroni and cheese is that you can play with with different cheeses that are equally tasty and melt well. Use Gruyère, Fontina, or smoked Gouda cheeses (or a combination).

Chapter Thirty-five

Chilli for manly men

Approximately 8 servings Time to Prepare: 25 minutes 1 hour and 15 minutes to prepare

Everything was new when we moved into our neighbourhood. There were new houses, a new school, new strip malls, and a new fire station in this newly built area. It was also the weekend of the Super Bowl. We invited our nice neighbours to come over, watch the game with us, and eat excessive amounts of chilli because we were such good neighbours. They agreed. The firefighters finished their chilli and asked for more. They raved about how delicious my chilli was because it was packed with beef, had a smoky taste, and was topped with bacon. I dubbed my meaty chilli Manly Man (firefighter-approved) Chili from then on.

2 tablespoons extra virgin olive oil

2 pound trimmed and sliced sirloin or round steak

1 pound Italian sausage, hot

1 big sliced onion

4 big minced garlic cloves

2 fire-roasted tomato cans (14.5 oz)

2 x 12-ounce beer bottles

2 8-ounce tomato sauce cans

a third cup of barbecue sauce (see Tips)

2 large green bell peppers, seeded and coarsely chopped (ribs removed).

2 large jalapeos, seeded and finely chopped (ribs removed).

chile powder (2 tablespoons)

4 tablespoons cumin powder

2 tablespoons coriander powder

2 teaspoons paprika (smoked)

2 teaspoons oregano, dried

12 teaspoon chilli powder

12 teaspoon black pepper, freshly ground

1 tablespoon salt

4 cups sharp cheddar cheese, shredded

sour cream, 2 cups

1 pound cooked and crumbled bacon (see Tips)

Heat the olive oil in a big, deep skillet over medium heat. Cook, tossing frequently to break up the steak and sausage, until it is cooked through and no longer pink, 6 to 8 minutes. Continue to stir and simmer for 1 minute after adding the garlic. Stir to incorporate the tomatoes, beer, tomato sauce, barbecue sauce, bell peppers, jalapeos, chilli powder, cumin, coriander, paprika, oregano, cayenne, black pepper, and salt. Bring the mixture to a boil, then lower the heat to a low setting. Cover the skillet and cook for 1 hour, or until the chilli has thickened. Serve in dishes with cheese, sour cream, and bacon crumbles on top.

ADAPTABLE WITHOUT GLUTEN Instead of beer, use 112 cups (gluten-free) beef broth. Make sure to use gluten-free barbecue sauce and bacon.

ADAPTABLE DAIRY-FREE Remove the sour cream and cheese.

TIPS The flavour of the chilli will be influenced by the barbecue sauce you choose. I prefer to use a sauce that has a smokey flavour.

Cook your bacon in the oven for simple cleanup. Preheat the oven to 400 degrees Fahrenheit. Place a rack on top of a big, rimmed baking sheet lined with foil. Using nonstick spray, coat the rack. On the rack, arrange the bacon strips. Bake for 15 to 20 minutes, or until crisp. The length of time depends on how thick your bacon is.

If you want to make this chilli more hotter, add another chopped jalapeo and boost the cayenne pepper to 12 tsp.

If you want to make a beef and bean chilli, add kidney or pinto beans to the mix.

Serve this chilli with a handful of corn chips on the side.

Chapter Thirty-six

Salad of grilled shrimp and vegetables with a lemon-basil dressing

Approximately 6 servings Time to Prepare: 25 minutes 12 minutes to prepare

Summer is the best season to make the most of fresh vegetables and barbecues. Do all of the chopping ahead of time for this one, and then toss everything together when you're ready to grill and serve. It's fantastic as a main dish salad or as a side dish salad with grilled meats.

SHRIMP WITH VEGETABLES

Peeled, deveined, and tails removed 112 pound big shrimp

2 medium red bell peppers, seeded and sliced into large chunks (ribs removed).

2 medium zucchini, cut ends and lengthwise sliced

2 tablespoons extra virgin olive oil

freshly ground black pepper and salt

VINAIGRETTE

3 tablespoons fresh basil, minced

2 1/2 tablespoons lemon juice, freshly squeezed

2 tablespoons extra virgin olive oil

2 minced medium garlic cloves

1 teaspoon white granulated sugar

1/2 teaspoon lemon zest, freshly grated

To taste, season with salt and freshly ground black pepper.

SALAD

6 cups greens (mixed)

Preheat your grill to medium.

Toss the shrimp and veggies with the olive oil and a generous sprinkling of salt and pepper in a medium mixing bowl. Place the shrimp and vegetables in a grill basket on top of the grill (see Tips). Grill the shrimp until they are pink, curled up, and cooked through, and the vegetables are softened and charred around the edges. Place the vegetables and shrimp on a cutting board. Transfer the shrimp and vegetables to a medium bowl and chop the vegetables into bite-size pieces.

SALAD OF GRILLED SHRIMP AND VEGETABLES WITH A...

To make the vinaigrette, whisk together all of the ingredients in a small bowl. Toss the shrimp and veggies in the vinaigrette to coat them. Cover the bowl with plastic wrap and keep it refrigerated if you are not serving the salad right away. Place the leaves in a large salad dish and top with the shrimp and veggies when ready to serve. Toss together and serve.

TIPS If you don't have a grill basket, throw the vegetables on the grill directly and skewer the shrimp for simple searing.

This salad can be prepared ahead of time. Because I love it cold, I grill the vegetables and shrimp first thing in the morning and let them marinate in the vinaigrette all day.

Instead of shrimp, use 112 pounds scallops or chicken (cut into bite-size pieces).

Chapter Thirty-seven

Broiled salmon with pineapple slaw

(sweet and spicy)

Serves 4 people Time to Prepare: 25 minutes 10 minutes to prepare

My sister, I believe, was the one who initially exposed me to the wonders of salmon. Of course, she lives in the Pacific Northwest, which has some of the greatest salmon I've ever had, prompting me to declare my love for it right then and there. Salmon is my go-to quick dinner to this day. I like it grilled and gently seasoned with a little additional sweetness, and it goes well with a simple sweet slaw.

SLAW

5 cups shredded cabbage (about 12 tiny heads)

12 cup canned pineapple, coarsely chopped (reserve 2 tablespoons juice for dressing)

SUPER CUTE RECIPES

1 medium red bell pepper, seeded, with ribs removed and thinly sliced

1 big peeled and shredded carrot

12 medium red onion, sliced very thinly (about 1 cup)

DRESSING

pineapple juice (two teaspoons) (from canned pineapples for slaw)

12 tbsp vegetable or canola oil

honey, 2 teaspoons

1 teaspoon lime juice, freshly squeezed

14 teaspoon cayenne pepper

1 teaspoon of salt

1/8 teaspoon black pepper, freshly ground

SALMON

4 skinless 6-ounce salmon fillets, rinsed and dried

a quarter-cup of honey

1 tablespoon lime juice, freshly squeezed

1 teaspoon cayenne pepper

cayenne pepper, 1/8 teaspoon

1 teaspoon of salt

To make the slaw, combine all of the ingredients in a large mixing dish.

To make the dressing, mix together the dressing ingredients in a small bowl.

Toss in the dressing with the slaw. Set aside the slaw while you finish the fish.

Preheat the broiler in the oven. Use nonstick spray to coat a small roasting pan or Pyrex dish.

Place the salmon in the pan to cook. Whisk together the honey, lime juice, chilli powder, cayenne, and salt in a small bowl. Pour the sauce over the salmon and serve. After 5 minutes of broiling, ladle the sauce over the salmon once more. Broil for 5 to 7 minutes more, or until the salmon flakes easily with a fork and is cooked through.

Toss the slaw one more time to incorporate the dressing before serving. Divide the slaw across four bowls. Serve the broiled salmon on top of the slaw right away.

MAKE-AHEAD SUGGESTIONS This recipe comes together quickly if all of the chopping and shredding is done ahead of time (up to 1 day). The dressing can also be made ahead of time and served the next day.

CPSIA information can be obtained
at www.ICGtesting.com
Printed in the USA
LVHW061604200722
723979LV00011B/173